BETTY BOOP'S

GUIDE TO A BOLD AND BALANCED LIFE

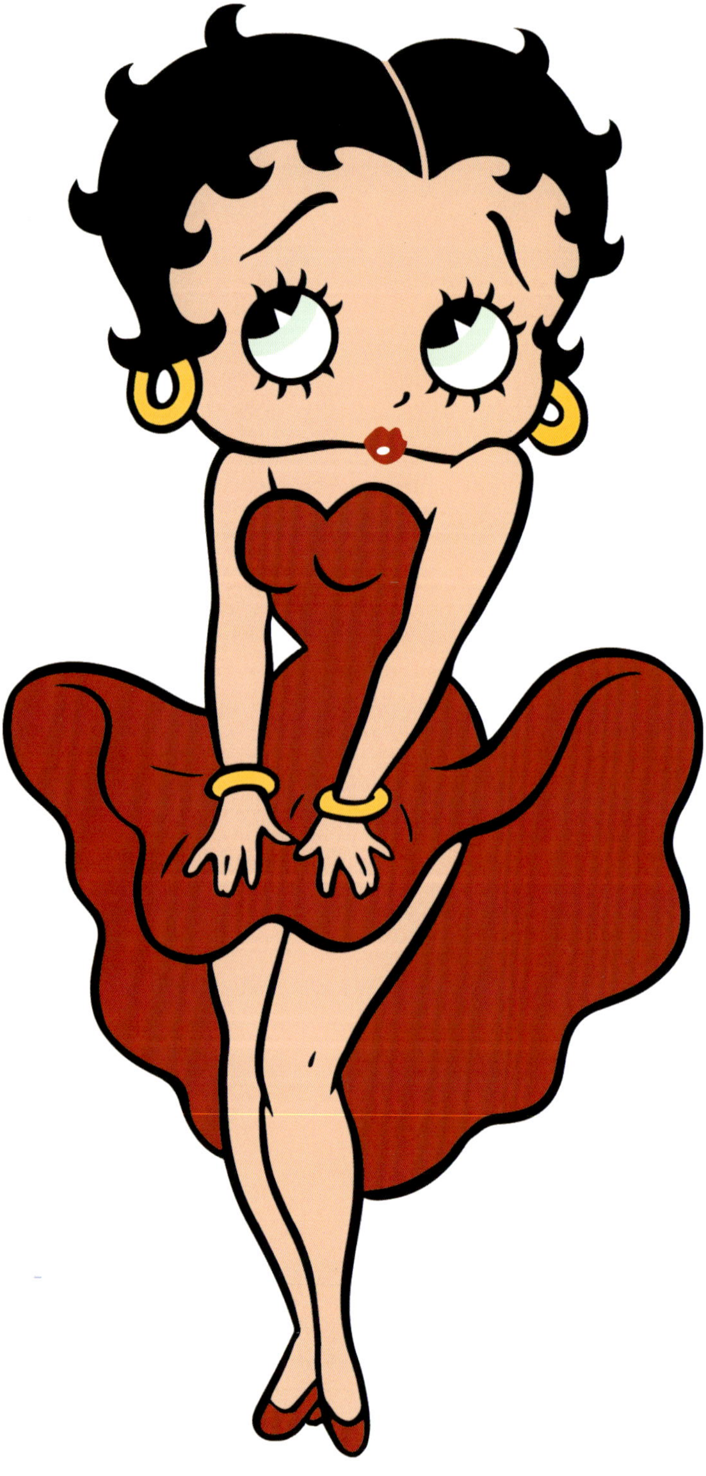

BETTY BOOP'S

GUIDE TO A BOLD AND BALANCED LIFE

FUN, FIERCE, FABULOUS ADVICE INSPIRED BY THE ANIMATED ICON

SUSAN WILKING HORAN
AND KRISTI LING SPENCER
with Betty Boop

Foreword by Zac Posen

Skyhorse Publishing

Skyhorse Publishing books may be purchased in bulk at special discounts for sales promotion, corporate gifts, fund-raising, or educational purposes. Special editions can also be created to specifications. For details, contact the Special Sales Department, Skyhorse Publishing, 307 West 36th Street, 11th Floor, New York, NY 10018 or info@skyhorsepublishing.com.

Skyhorse® and Skyhorse Publishing® are registered trademarks of Skyhorse Publishing, Inc.®, a Delaware corporation.

Visit our website at www.skyhorsepublishing.com.

10 9 8 7 6 5 4 3 2 1

Library of Congress Cataloging-in-Publication Data is available on file.

Cover design by Daniel Brount

Print ISBN: 978-1-5107-5005-0
Ebook ISBN: 978-1-5107-5008-1

Printed in China

Authors' Note: The content of this book is a compilation of our own research and experience with advice and tips supported by scientific evidence and, of course, inspired by the indomitable Betty Boop. This information is intended to help readers make informed decisions about their lifestyle habits in an educational and entertaining way. As always, before changing any aspect of one's lifestyle, including medical, diet, fitness and exercise programs, career or relationship paths, one should always consult first with one's own experienced team of mental and physical health care advisors and professionals. Nothing in this book is designed to be a substitute for the treatment or advice received from one's own doctor or primary care physician. And, of course, in the event the information or advice within this book differs from information or advice provided by health care community experts, readers should always follow the recommendation of those experts.

Contents

Foreword by Zac Posen *vii*

Introduction *1*

Chapter 1: Embrace Your Independence 5

Chapter 2: Love Is All You Need 30

Chapter 3: A Little Kindness Goes a Long Way 48

Chapter 4: Going in Style 64

Chapter 5: Accentuate the Positive 84

Chapter 6: Cultivating Courage 100

Chapter 7: Confidence: The Must-Have Accessory 122

Chapter 8: Humor Makes the World Go 'Round 138

Chapter 9: Health—Our Ultimate Wealth 160

Chapter 10: Respect-fully Yours 186

That's a Wrap! *206*

Acknowledgments *210*

About the Authors *211*

Foreword

I've always been a huge fan of Betty's. She has been a part of my life since I was a child and I have always seen her as a social icon who has navigated the changing times and styles through the decades. As one of the earliest female superwomen to enter the comic and animation spectrum, Betty is a reflection of women's history and their path to Independence.

I am all about women with ambition and drive, and Betty exudes both. She forged her path to Independence along with other great women of her time, including Amelia Earhart and Florence Nightingale. Betty's entire career as an animated character has paralleled the real-life struggles and challenges of real women everywhere. Let's face it—women have always had to work harder to be successful and to be taken seriously. They have to be strong, determined, and unwilling to give up when it comes to making their dreams come true.

Over the course of the ninety years she's been around, Betty has seen it all and she's done it all. She's been a nurse, school teacher, judge, automotive mechanic, and hotel proprietor. She's sung and danced with the greats, including Cab Calloway, Louis Armstrong, and Ethel Merman. She was an outspoken supporter of animal rights long before it became a celebrated cause, and in 1932 Betty even ran for president! The very first female—animated or not—to enter that political arena. She embodies the concepts of ambition, resilience, and longevity.

She's had her ups and downs and has been through huge moments that have made history such as Prohibition, the Industrial Revolution, the Great Depression, the Technological Age, and even a brand-new century, just to name a few. But she takes everything she experiences, learns from it, and becomes a better person *because* of it. I love that life never seems to get Betty down. She always manages to rise to the occasion, handling everything with grace and humor.

Betty exudes style—not just in the dress she wears—but in the warmth, humor, confidence, and compassion she shows to everyone and everything around her. She has the ability to change as the world around her changes. And through it all, she ultimately has grown into not only the best version of herself, but also an immortal role model throughout time. Her message that *no matter what, stay true to yourself, keep believing in your dreams, pursue your goals, and never give up* will never die and will always be a significant sentiment shared with women everywhere.

I know that Betty will live on forever!

ZAC POSEN, celebrated fashion designer

Introduction

Welcome to *Betty Boop's Guide to a Bold and Balanced Life*! We're so happy to have you join us on this fun, inspiring, and uniquely entertaining journey. As two women who are enthusiastic advocates for women's health, happiness, and empowerment—and who also have worked with Betty Boop and her parent company Fleischer Studios for many years—we knew we could bring this much-needed book to life in a thoughtful, colorful, and big way for Betty's fans and women everywhere.

This is the first book of its kind that speaks directly to the millions of women who over the years have been moved by Betty's empowering persona. It's the first in which the details of Betty, her history, her defeats, her victories, and the lessons she has learned from her travels through time are shared with her friends and fans. It's the perfect opportunity for all of us to spend a little more time with our favorite animated screen star. And, whether you've been a lifelong fan of Betty's or have just recently been introduced to her, we know you'll have a great time getting to know her even better within the pages of this book.

INSPIRATION FROM BETTY

As one of the most popular animated characters of all time, Betty Boop is beloved by women of all ages around the world in part because of her adorable appearance, her friendly accessibility, and her signature phrase, "Boop-Oop-a-Doop." But she also is adored because of her enchanting wit, humor, inspiring messages, and ahead-of-her-time wisdom.

After all, there's a little bit of Betty in each of us. When you watch her classic cartoons, scroll her social media feeds, or just read about the powerful ways she's influenced society and pop culture over the decades, there's something about Betty we can all relate to. Ambitious, vibrant, and confident, she seeks to make a positive change in the world around her. She's sassy, classy, and full of moxie. She's stylish and flirty. A no-nonsense girl, she's proud of who she is and won't apologize for it. She's been through some tough times and come out stronger. And, she's definitely a girl we'd all like to hang out with—an experience we've tried to create for you in this book!

TOPICS WE'LL BE CHATTING ABOUT

Now, there are *many* topics we could talk about when it comes to Betty's great adventures and her daring approach to life. Her harrowing, inspiring, and empowering experiences over the years are still so relevant in the lives of women today. And there are several topics we could discuss that are so important in this world of countless challenges and complications. We have carefully selected ten universal themes that have always been cornerstones for Betty's life, and remain so for all women striving to create the beautiful, bold, and balanced life we all desire and deserve.

Pulled directly from the classic Betty Boop cartoons specifically for this book, we'll be covering the topics of Independence, Love, Kindness, Style, Positivity, Courage, Confidence, Humor, Health, and Respect.

In each chapter you'll find gems of wisdom, super helpful advice, and amusing and engaging stories from Betty's life that everyone can relate to. You'll also find a wonderful blend of important messages, problem-solving tips, humorous anecdotes, fascinating scientific studies, and practical information for making every day your best.

You'll learn how to handle difficult situations, boost your brain power, improve your health, bolster your relationships, minimize your weaknesses, and maximize your strengths. And you'll do it all with a little help from Betty!

Finally, of course, we've filled these pages with adorable images of Betty—both old and new—to showcase her journey, illustrate her timeless lessons, and demonstrate her innate ability to evolve with and adjust to the ever-changing world around her. After all, what would a book inspired by our favorite sass symbol be without a ton of fabulous animated photos?

And, all of this we've done with the intent of creating a unique, personal, intimate, and one-of-a-kind reading experience we hope you'll absolutely love!

THE BEST WAY TO ENJOY THIS BOOK

We've purposely packed this book with helpful, inspiring, and universally recognized tips and advice of all kinds. So, whether you've heard some of it before, or it's completely new to you, the best way to enjoy this particular book is to just dive in, be open to new experiences, and get ready for a good time!

One thing you'll learn quickly as you begin to read, is that Betty loves lists! She loves to write things down because doing so helps her to remember details and to focus on things important to her. So, you may want to have some paper or a journal close by, a highlighter, and a few pencils and pens. These will also prove to be handy tools when we ask you to join us in a helpful exercise or two.

We also encourage you to dog-ear pages and underline! You may find yourself wanting to read a few sections twice when something you read makes you smile, tugs at your soul, or like Betty's Grampy—illuminates that light bulb over your head. It's time to relax, light a candle, pour a glass of your favorite beverage, and enjoy.

And once you begin this journey with Betty and us, invite your friends to join the party! It's a lot easier—and a lot more fun—to travel a new path and learn new lessons when you do it with those you love. So, phone, text, tweet, post, and share *Betty Boop's Guide* to your heart's content. Help us spread the fun! After all, the more the merrier. And, everyone can use a little inspiration!

A LITTLE MORE ABOUT BETTY

If there's one thing Betty knows, it's how to make a lasting impression. For more than ninety years, the glamorous international icon has sung, sashayed, and "Boop-Oop-a-Dooped" past rules and conventions, unafraid to take risks or set trends, and proving time after time that she can do anything she sets her mind to.

First introduced in 1930, Betty Boop was created by Max Fleischer for his "Talkartoons" series, the first "talkies" of animation, which Max's company,

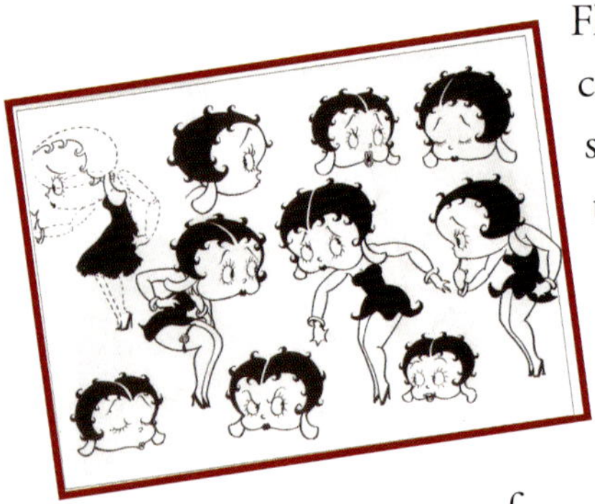

Fleischer Studios, produced for Paramount. By 1932 Betty, considered to be the first and only female animated screen star, had taken the country by storm. She starred in more than 100 cartoons, 90 of which are included in the official *Betty Boop* series, which ended in 1939.

Since then, Betty has appeared in dozens of hit movies, television specials, and commercials. She was the first cartoon character to be profiled by A&E's famous *Biography* series. Her popularity today shines through her prevalence in pop culture. A media darling and fashion icon, she appears on everything from T-shirts to cosmetics to high-fashion designs. It's hard to go very long without spotting Betty *somewhere*.

OUR GOAL FOR YOU

Our goal is that you'll not only enjoy reading this book, but that you'll be able to use the helpful tips and advice inspired by this beloved character to bring more joy, boldness, and balance into your life and the lives of those you love. We all deserve to live our very best lives, and it's definitely helpful to have a little inspiration and support along the way—especially when it can be this much fun!

We know your choices are many and we extend you a huge *thank-you* for picking up this book! We're so glad you're here! We hope you have as much fun reading this book as we did writing it for you. It's been a grand adventure and we're so grateful for the opportunity to share it. We look forward to connecting with you through our websites and social media—because we wrote this book for *you*—and we're so excited to know what you think!

Sending much love and Betty magic,
KRISTI AND SUSAN

Chapter 1

Embrace Your Independence

One of the most beloved classic animated characters in the world, Betty Boop was created in 1930 by the legendary pioneer animator, Max Fleischer. Like many of us, Betty's life journey has taken many unexpected twists and turns over the years. In fact, when Betty was first introduced by Max and his company, Fleischer Studios, her character and appearance were a combination of human and canine characteristics. After all, she had a supporting role as a singer in a night club run and frequented by hip music-loving dogs!

Betty became so popular, however, that she soon took center stage and over time she evolved into the spunky, confident, and outspoken character we know today. Her face became softer and undeniably human. Her dog-like ears became her trademark hoop earrings. Her feminine figure, colorful garter, bangle bracelet, and tiny, high-heeled shoes became synonymous with the image and emergence of the strong-willed, independent woman of the twentieth century.

Since her beginning, Betty Boop has entertained millions of adoring fans and inspired legions of women with her self-reliant, spirited, empowered persona. In her animated films, Betty stood up to bullies, fought for animal rights, advocated for health and happiness, refused to tolerate harassment of any kind, and even ran for president of the United States. No wonder she sassed, sang, and sashayed her way into the hearts of so many!

One of Betty's most notable and admirable traits is her independence. She is perfectly happy as a single woman, goes after what she wants, and rises to take on any challenge that comes her way. So naturally, the topic of independence is the perfect way to kick off this book!

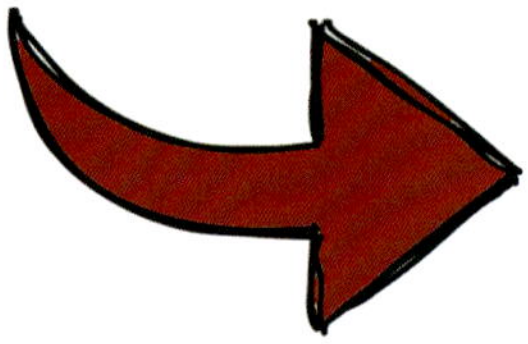

What Exactly Is Independence and What Does It Mean to Be Independent?

Well, if we look to *Merriam-Webster*, the term "Independent" means:

1. Being *not* dependent.
2. Not subject to control by others.
3. Not requiring or relying on something else.
4. Not looking to others for one's opinions or for guidance in conduct.

And, if we take all these definitions together, we have an ideal that no animated character in the world embodies better or more completely than the iconic Betty Boop.

From her very beginnings, Betty has been a trailblazer extraordinaire! Through several decades she remains sassy, confident, strong, *and* an amazing example of what it means to be independent for today's woman in today's world.

Because, let's face it. Women have never had it easy. Women have always had to work harder than their male counterparts to be successful and taken seriously. To be noticed and recognized. To support themselves and their families and to earn equal pay in the workplace.

For years, many strong, independent, free-thinking women have sacrificed and struggled to pave the way for today's woman—the modern woman.

And, no one—certainly no one in the animated world—can trace this path to independence like Betty Boop. Through her decades-long career as a screen siren, spokesperson, social icon, and cultural commentator, the animated history of Betty Boop has paralleled the real-life history of women everywhere. Women who are trying to find themselves. Women who are trying to make a difference by taking chances and striving every day to transform their dreams into reality.

Because, while we have not lived through the changes of the last hundred years—our mothers, grandmothers, and great grandmothers have. And, right next to them in the middle of the fight was our Betty. Her story is a reflection of our country's history, our personal history, and of women's history.

So, with Betty's help let's get our Boop-Oop-a-Doop on and take a trip down memory lane—exploring the evolution of the modern woman and her road to independence.

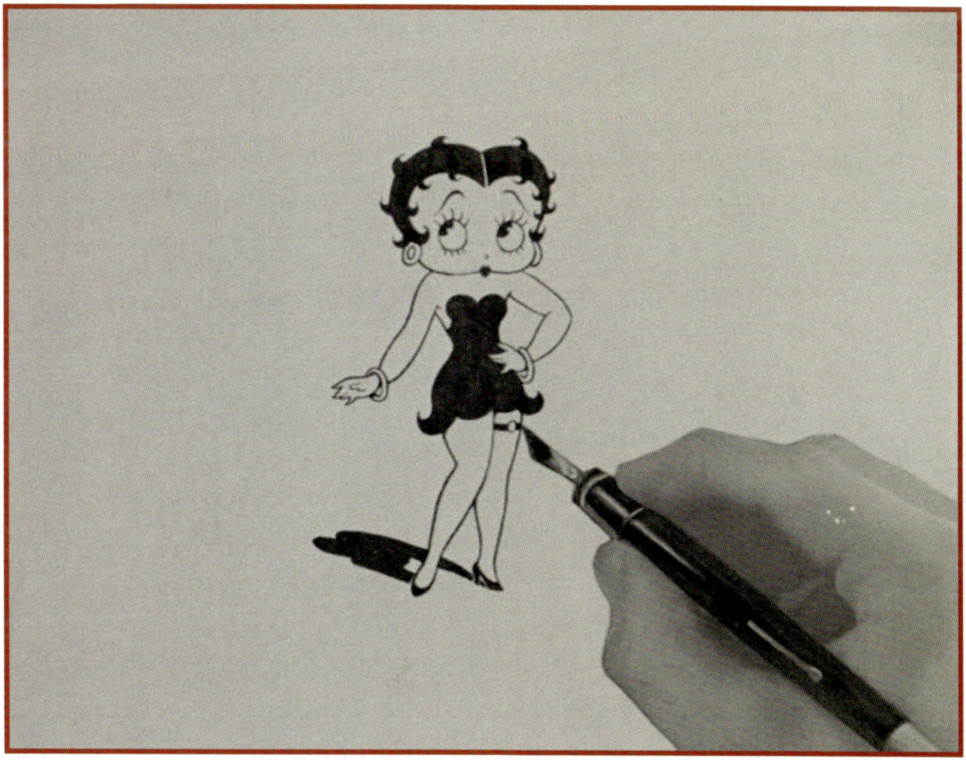

THE PRINCIPLE– Getting to Know Yourself

Betty's Inspiration: Before we can be independent, we need to know who we are and what we want.

Keep a Journal of Your Daily Activities. At the end of each day, reflect on your entries. Ask yourself what activities made you feel calm, happy, or satisfied, and what activities made you feel agitated, stressed, or worried.

Meet Your Own Needs. Once you begin to identify those things in your life that please you, add more to your schedule. In contrast, reduce the time you spend on activities that create stress. Learn to recognize what you like, need, and want in life—and then act accordingly. If you're lonely, call up a friend. If you're tired, go home and get an early night.

Become More Assertive. As you become more aware of your likes and dislikes, learn to say "yes" and "no." As simple as this sounds, assertiveness is a powerful skill. Set healthy boundaries for yourself. Only say "yes" when you mean it. And, say "no" whenever you have doubts about a situation or a commitment. Don't force yourself to do anything with which you're uncomfortable.

Respect Your Emotions. Give yourself permission to feel your changing emotions. Acknowledge sadness and confusion as much as you acknowledge joy and confidence. Determine the cause of each emotion. Understand that each is a normal reaction. Know that each is temporary in nature. And, move on with your day.

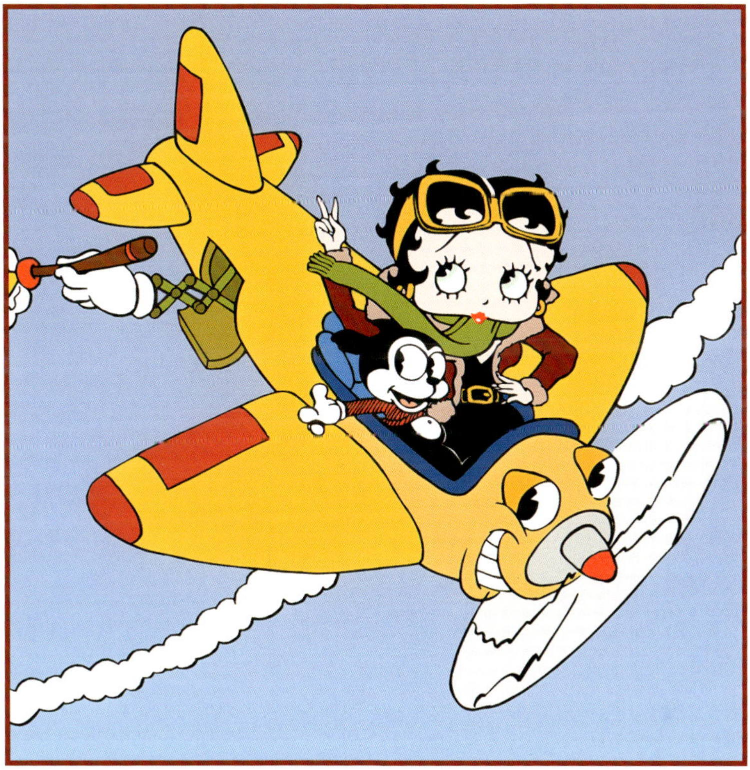

Getting to know ourselves in this way is the basis of "autonomy." And autonomy is essential for developing Independence and decreasing dependence.

Just look at Betty. She is the essence of American autonomy. She knows who she is and what she wants. She is the author of her own life. She writes the rules by which she lives. She owns her own opinions, thoughts, feelings, and perceptions. She has developed the confidence to be herself and so can you!

Yet, developing autonomy and independence *is a process*. Especially for women. And, no time in history was a better example of this than . . .

THE PROGRESSIVE ERA IN AMERICA

From about 1890 to about 1920 the positions of power in American society were typically held by men. Men were the politicians, landowners, storekeepers, entrepreneurs, business leaders, and decision-makers.

Women, on the other hand, were limited to the roles of housekeepers, mothers, and wives. It was extremely difficult for women to work outside the home. Basically, women were dependent on husbands or parents for their support. Why? Because most women still lacked a higher education and job skills.

Fortunately, there were three careers for women for which they could train and find work. And, Betty has been them all!

The first was to be a nurse. Thanks to the independent work and dedication of Florence Nightingale in the late 1800s, this occupation was elevated from lowly menial labor to the honorable and respected vocation it is today.

The field of nursing opened the first career doors for many women giving them the chance to venture outside the home and engage in meaningful and important work. It also allowed women to join the fight and lend their voices to the cause when America entered World War I in 1917.

> "I ATTRIBUTE MY SUCCESS TO THIS—I NEVER GAVE OR TOOK ANY EXCUSE."
>
> —FLORENCE NIGHTINGALE, MOTHER OF MODERN NURSING

The second career was that of a seamstress. You see, clothing manufacturing was big business at the beginning of the twentieth century. And, factory owners *loved* hiring women—not to mention children—because they could pay them lower wages than those paid to men. And sewing, after all, was "women's work."

And, the third career option was to become a school teacher. In fact, it was the inclusion of women into this noble profession that brought about much-needed reform in the fields of child psychology, welfare, and education. This female presence not only improved education for children, but also enabled more women to enter the world of higher education themselves.

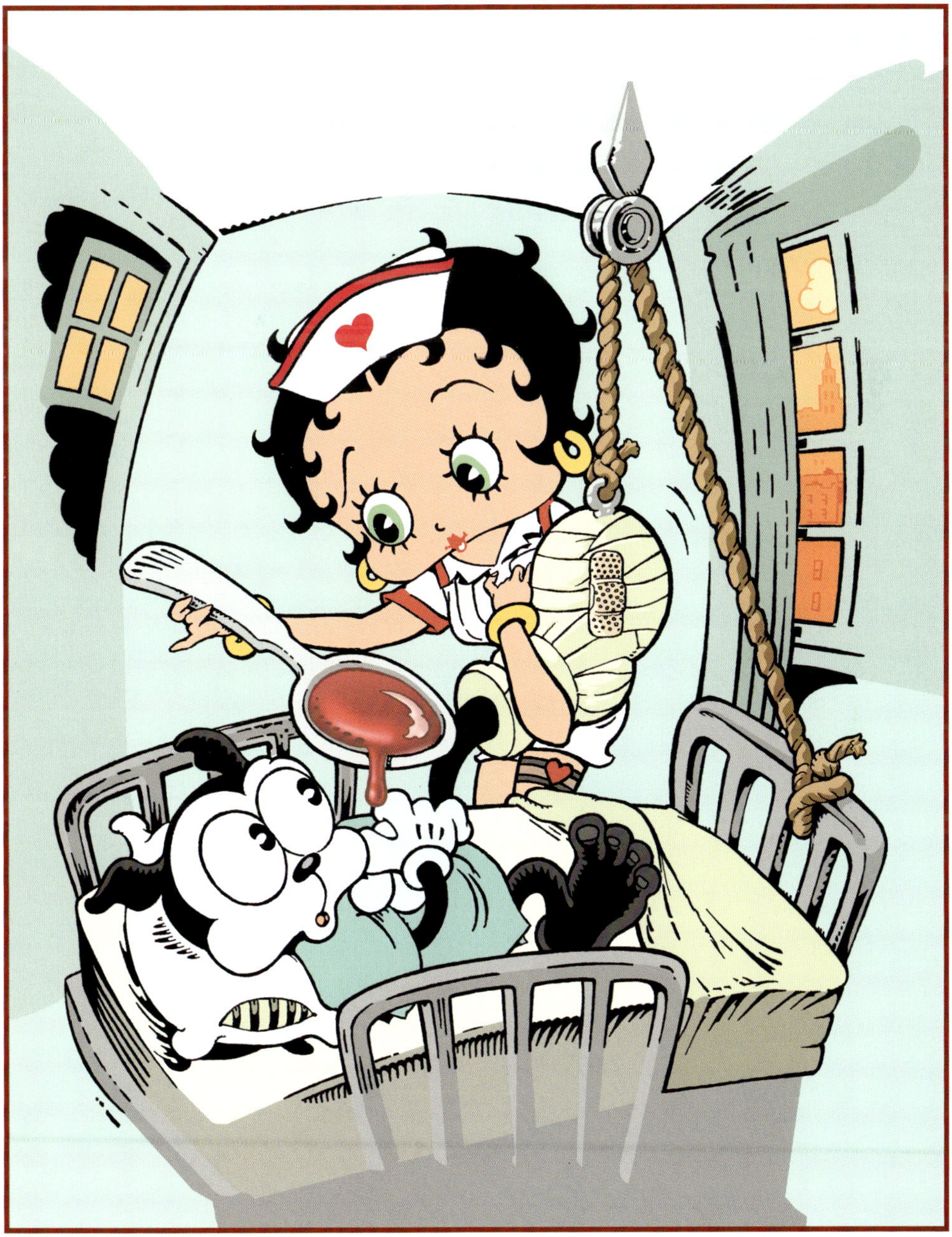

Of course, a huge part of being independent is having a career and the ability to provide for ourselves. Fortunately, women today can become *anything* they want. So, the difficulty is not in having limited career options—the difficulty today is in trying to decide on one career from an unlimited field of possibilities.

THE PRINCIPLE– Choosing a Career

Betty's Inspiration: With the luxury of choice today, be sure the career you pick is just right for you.

Determine Where Your Interests Lie. This, of course, is a big part of getting to know yourself. And, you've already started to work on that. So, now it's time to expand your knowledge a bit. Do you have a passion? Do you love animals? Are you good at math? Do you like taking care of others? What are your values? Do you prefer being indoors or outdoors? Make a list of the things at which you excel or simply enjoy.

Do Your Research. Set aside thirty minutes each day. During this time comb through Internet career sites, read business blogs that you like, and scan top job rankings or "help wanted" sections of the newspaper. Keep a list of the jobs that catch your eye and pique your interest.

Get Help from the Experts. You now have a list of your interests and a list of jobs that appeal to you. It's time to contact a professional who can help you find a few good matches. Talk to a career counselor at your local college or university. Make an appointment with a career development facilitator. Check with the local libraries, which typically offer career planning services free of charge. Explore the options together. Fresh eyes are always helpful!

Understand Your Priorities. Are you willing to relocate for your job? Does your work have to be important to the world? Do you just want to make good money?

Are you willing to start at the bottom and work your way up? Do you need a comfortable environment or can you work anywhere? Decide what's important to you.

Make Your Best-Informed Decision. Eventually, you have to make a decision. But remember, your responsibility is to make an informed decision based on your best evidence and research at the time. Nothing is written in stone. If your first or second or even third choice doesn't work out, you'll find something else. It's all a learning process.

Thank goodness women today have choices when it comes to their career. We enjoy the luxury of choosing from a deep pool of possibilities, when our female predecessors didn't.

Yet, women at the turn of the last century did realize that *when they bonded together as nurses, seamstresses, teachers, wives, and mothers, they created a powerful voice for social change.*

Women began calling themselves "municipal housekeepers" instead of homemakers to gain entrance into community affairs. They strived to "clean up" and create social reform in education, politics, public health, and state welfare.

First, our early female activists formed the Women's Suffrage Movement. Because, there was a time when women weren't even allowed to vote! *Can you imagine?!*

Our Sister Suffragettes worked for decades to pass the Nineteenth Amendment, which in 1920 finally gave women the right to vote. Hooray! That's one for the girls!

> "WOMAN MUST NOT DEPEND UPON THE PROTECTION OF MAN, BUT MUST BE TAUGHT TO PROTECT HERSELF."
>
> —SUSAN B. ANTHONY, SUFFRAGETTE AND WOMEN'S RIGHTS ACTIVIST

"Lips that touch wine shall never touch mine."

Second, women tackled the issue of Prohibition. Okay, for those who may not be familiar with this 1920s phenomenon, Prohibition was the law that made the production, transportation, and sale of liquor and alcoholic beverages illegal.

Led by concerned women known as THE TEMPERANCE LEAGUE, this law was not passed because women were against the use of alcohol—rather, it was passed because the working husbands and fathers of these women typically spent their payday at the end of each week in bars and saloons spending their paycheck on liquid entertainment. As a result, hard-earned money often would be gone before these men even returned home.

And this, of course, meant the women—their wives, mothers, and sisters—had no means with which to feed their families. As a result, women joined together again and succeeded in passing Prohibition—a constitutional ban that remained in effect for more than a decade.

And third, women began to challenge the Victorian values of the time that encouraged men to dominate wage work and politics while keeping women in the sphere of domestic work and childrearing.

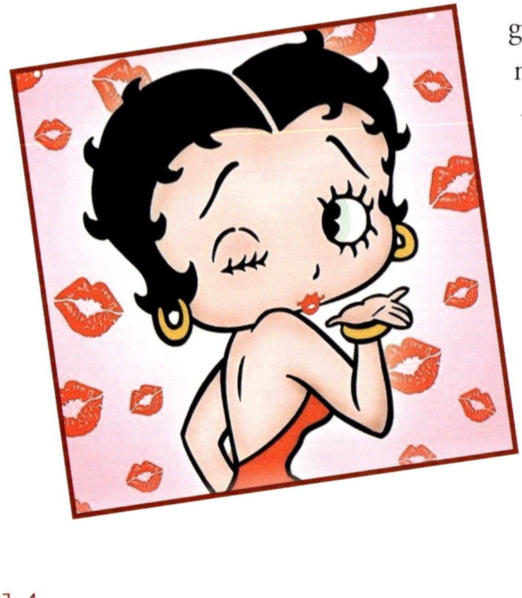

Under the pressure of Women Progressives—especially the young, single, middle-class women working in the cities—these paradigms began to change and society was forced to reinvent itself once again.

THE PRINCIPLE– Blaze Your Own Trail

Betty's Inspiration: Just because something hasn't been done before doesn't mean it can't be done.

Be Willing to Take Risks. There is an adage which says, "If you want things to be different, you have to do things differently." This means taking chances. It means thinking outside the box. And, it means taking action without a guarantee of the outcome.

Stretch Your Comfort Zone. Blazing a new trail and trying something different can be uncomfortable. And, it can be scary. So, every day do at least one thing that makes you uncomfortable. Push the envelope as they say, but do it gently.

Make Necessary Sacrifices. Getting something always requires giving something. Be prepared to make a few sacrifices of time, money, or leisure activities to get where you want to be.

Celebrate the Wins. Blazing a new trail takes time. It doesn't happen overnight. It's a process of small victories. So, make sure to pat yourself on the back with every small success you achieve. You deserve it!

Thanks to the Women Progressives, the 1920s was an age of dramatic political and social change which, indeed, earned this decade the nickname of . . .

THE ROARING TWENTIES

People were moving to urban areas and becoming "city slickers." America was experiencing great economic growth and began its love affair with the automobile. Of course, with the creation of the car came freedom. And, it was this environment into which the New Woman was born.

Known as "flappers," these were the fashionistas of the time—the women who made heads turn and made headlines!

What's more, women now were commonly employed in business as stenographers, shop keepers, and secretaries. Birth control devices such as the diaphragm allowed women to choose the number of children they wanted, or whether to have children at all. And, new technology helped eliminate the drudgery of housework and free up more time for women to expand in creative and innovative ways.

So, with these modern technologies and new-found freedoms came the beginning of . . .

THE JAZZ AGE

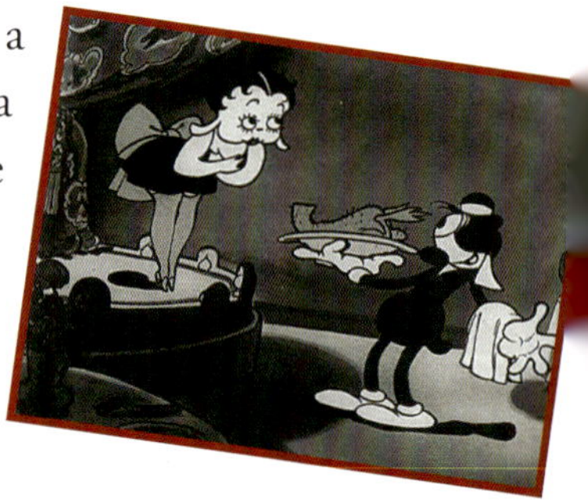

And, our Betty was a part of it all. First appearing as a singer in a night club, Betty evolved from a singing quasi-dog character to a full-fledged singing female human character. She epitomized the women's movement of the Roaring Twenties and into the 1930s with her fierce Independence and resolve to stand up for herself.

The music sizzled and Betty brought her own sass—and just a bit of crass—to perform with jazz greats like Cab Calloway, Louis Armstrong, Ethel Merman, The Mills Brothers, Don Redman, and the big-voiced Mary Small.

Betty and the women of the time took the baton from their predecessors—women like Florence Nightingale and Susan B. Anthony—and ran confidently with it into the future. Betty was not only a part of it, but in many ways led the charge!

MOVING THROUGH THE THIRTIES

However, the road to Independence for women was about to hit a roadblock. When the Great Depression engulfed America, approximately 12 million people were out of work.

So once again, women were discouraged from entering the work force and "taking" jobs away from men. In fact, some states passed laws forbidding employers from hiring women at all! *Yet, women kept fighting and following their dreams.*

> "THE MOST EFFECTIVE WAY TO DO IT, IS TO DO IT!"
> –AMELIA EARHART, AVIATION PIONEER AND AUTHOR

Amelia Earhart became the first female aviator to fly solo across the Atlantic Ocean.

And, Betty Boop—one female who was never satisfied with the status quo—ran for president! That's right! Even though women now had the right to vote, in 1932 Betty decided it was time for a woman to become president.

In the classic cartoon *Betty Boop for President*, Betty tackles politics and pokes a bit of fun at those on both sides of the aisle. In part, Betty strove to lighten the depressed mood of the country and in part, she was making a satirical comment on the state of American politics.

I can do anything a man can do!
Don't be a Poop. Vote for Boop!

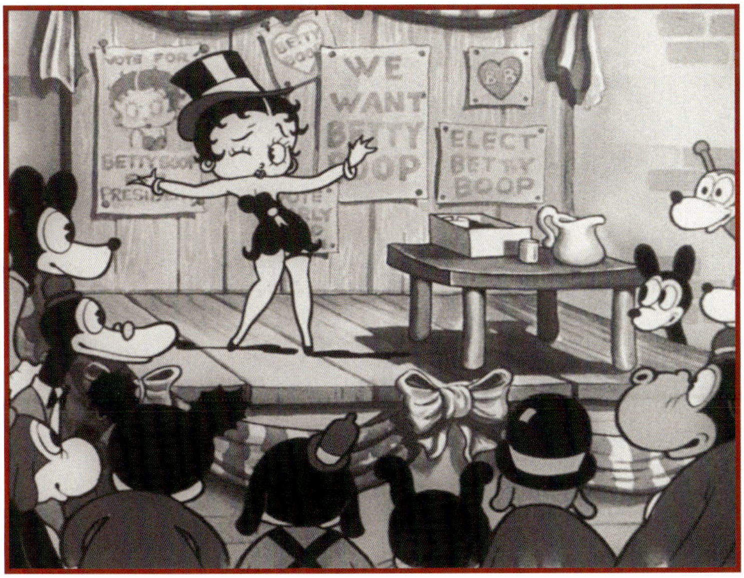

THE PRINCIPLE–
Dream Big

Betty's Inspiration: Always remember, everything begins with a dream.

A Dream Can Never Be Too Big. Dreaming is a huge part of who we are. It's within our dreams that we learn to fly without limitations. Don't put boundaries on your desires or abilities. If your dream doesn't scare you, it's probably not big enough. Anything is possible!

Take Action. A dream will only become reality if you act on it. And for every action you take, push yourself to do a little bit more. Work an hour later. Write one extra blog post. Take that weekend seminar. It's up to *you* to make your dreams come true.

Seek Inspiration from Others. Surround yourself with others who also dream big. Be inspired by those who never take no for an answer. Learn from their experience. Read about the successes and failures of those you admire. Follow their example of never giving up. Dreaming is contagious!

Follow Your Heart. Be true to yourself. You know yourself better than anyone else. Don't cave in to outside pressure. Don't listen to those who say you can't. Stay the course and think for yourself. Use your inner compass and be your own True North!

Don't Be Afraid to Make Mistakes. The only person who never makes a mistake is the person who never tries. Reaching your goals and becoming successful will be a process of trial and error. We learn from our mistakes. They are an important part of developing independence and making our dreams come true.

Betty Boop for President was released on November 4, four days before the 1932 Presidential election. It was an interesting social precursor as the economic emergency of the 1930s led to significant political gains for women.

For one, the New Deal, a social welfare package, led to the appointment of more women in high government positions. And, these women used their new government posts to work on behalf of other women! How great is that?!

"THE FIRST, LAST, AND MAIN THING PEOPLE WANT AND HAVE A RIGHT TO IS A JOB."

–MOLLY DEWSON, REFORMER AND NEW DEAL POLITICAL ACTIVIST

Not everyone, however, appreciated the fact that women were becoming more independent and were flexing their freedom muscles in far-reaching new ways. Women—even animated women—had to keep fighting for their rights and independence.

When a little censorship device called The Hays Code a.k.a. The Motion Picture Production Code was enacted in 1930 to "clean up" the entertainment industry, Betty Boop was forced to change her attitude and appearance. Her dress became long-skirted and high-necked. Her garter disappeared. And, her attitude became demure and subservient.

But, not for long! Betty had her own way of protesting! In *A Language All My Own* Betty sang to a Japanese audience in both English and Japanese. And, while the English version was "squeaky clean" and Hays Code-approved, the Japanese version contained a few phrases the Code would never have approved. Betty was always fighting for the right to exercise her independence—and speak for herself!

THE PRINCIPLE– Stand Up for Yourself

Betty's Inspiration: The ability to express yourself honestly will change the way other people see you and the way you see yourself.

Clarify Your Needs and Wants. When facing an uncomfortable situation, write down your feelings. Determine the cause of your discomfort.

Create a Script. If you are facing a confrontation, figure out what you want to say *before* you speak. Be honest and assertive. Write down your thoughts. Include phrases like, "I feel uncomfortable about this because . . ." or "I disagree because . . ." or "I would rather do it this way because . . ." Be respectful of others but be clear about your feelings. Following a script is easier and more effective than winging it in a difficult conversation.

Practice Saying No. Sometimes saying "no" is all we have to do to stand our ground. Most of us say "yes" out of politeness and a fear of hurting the feelings of others. Begin by saying "no" in non-critical situations. In time, you will be able to speak up for yourself in any situation.

Own Your Victories. Standing up for yourself can be hard. As women, many of us were raised to smile, be sweet, and say, "yes." Changing this behavior will take time. So, be sure to congratulate yourself every time you stand your ground and speak up. Small steps lead to big changes!

RACING THROUGH THE CENTURY

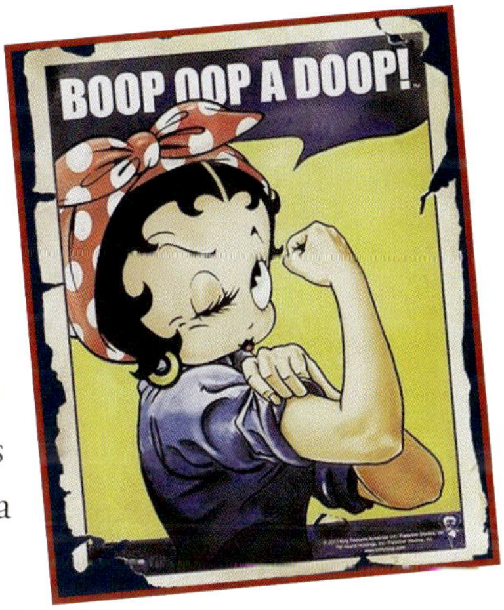

Women's Independence reached new heights in the 1940s as war once again engulfed the world. Women joined the labor force and filled the jobs enlisted men left vacant.

The Women's Army Corp (WAC) and the Women Accepted for Volunteer Emergency Services (WAVES) were both established. And, the All-American Girls Professional Baseball League was founded! Talk about a home run!

Throughout the next few decades, women entered the work place in droves. And, the progress of women during the 1940s and 1950s laid the groundwork for the Feminist Movement of the 1960s and 1970s.

Brave Independent women challenged racial bias and pushed for civil rights reform.

> "I WOULD HAVE TO KNOW ONCE AND FOR ALL WHAT RIGHTS I HAD AS A HUMAN BEING AND A CITIZEN."
> –ROSA PARKS, ACTIVIST AND MOTHER OF THE FREEDOM MOVEMENT

Motivated women everywhere focused on dismantling workplace inequality and establishing the Equal Rights Amendment. And, just as Betty fought off unwanted advances by a lecherous circus ringmaster in 1932's *Boop-Oop-a-Doop*, women of the 1960s and 1970s began the long fight against sexual harassment in the workplace.

THE PRINCIPLE– Dealing with Harassment

Betty's Inspiration: Knowing how to protect yourself in the workplace is an essential skill in today's world.

Create a Paper Trail. Immediately record the name of the person harassing you, the date, the location, the time, and a description of the event. Documentation is important!

Get Witnesses. Consult with your fellow coworkers. Ask if they have had the same problem. If anyone sees the event, ask them to make a record and write it down. If you're being harassed, the chances are good that others are as well. There is safety in numbers.

Try to Keep Calm. As upsetting as harassment is, don't act when you are in a state of emotional turmoil. Collect yourself and your thoughts. When you are calm you are more articulate and professional. You are better able to present your case.

Report to a Supervisor. Gather your written evidence, your witnesses, and meet with your boss or supervisor. If your boss or supervisor is the one responsible for the harassment, contact your human resources representative.

Always Follow Up. If your complaints fall on deaf ears, talk to higher management. Sexual harassment is against the law. Even bullying can be a form of employment discrimination or assault, both of which are illegal. If necessary and as a last resort, explore your legal options inside *and* outside your place of employment.

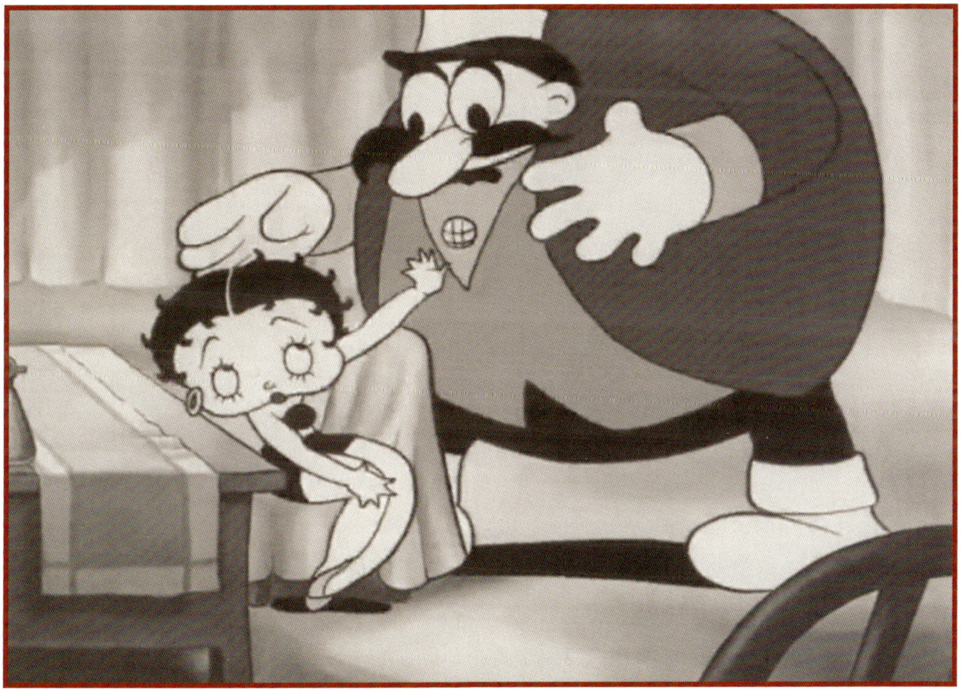

INDEPENDENCE IN THE MODERN WORLD

Yep—women have fought hard for the rights, privileges, and freedoms we enjoy today. It hasn't been an easy process. It hasn't happened quickly and it's certainly not over.

Many of the issues women faced a century ago are still being faced by women today—even animated women like Betty Boop. We still have to work hard, speak loudly, step firmly, stick up for ourselves, and fight the occasional battle.

Nevertheless, we have come so far! And, no one has been a part of this incredible transformation and marvelous march to Independence longer than Betty Boop. Which means, as we plant our feet firmly in the twenty-first century there's no one more qualified than Betty to remind us of all we've accomplished!

Women Today Can Vote

Remember, this basic right was difficult to obtain and it took our Sister Suffragettes decades to deliver. In fact, the right to vote has become so instilled in our modern culture that it's considered unacceptable when we don't vote!

Women Today Are Involved in Politics and Government

We are becoming senators, congresswomen, judges, mayors, and governors. And, these platforms allow women to effect more positive and inclusive change in the world around us.

Women Today Have Choices

Women have the freedom to *choose* what they want to do for a living. We hold jobs and positions that traditionally were reserved for men.

We can do things we've never done before *or* we can do things we've always done before! Today when we become mothers, family caregivers, wives, and homemakers, it's not because others tell us we can't do anything else. It's because we *love* these roles and we *choose* to work in the home.

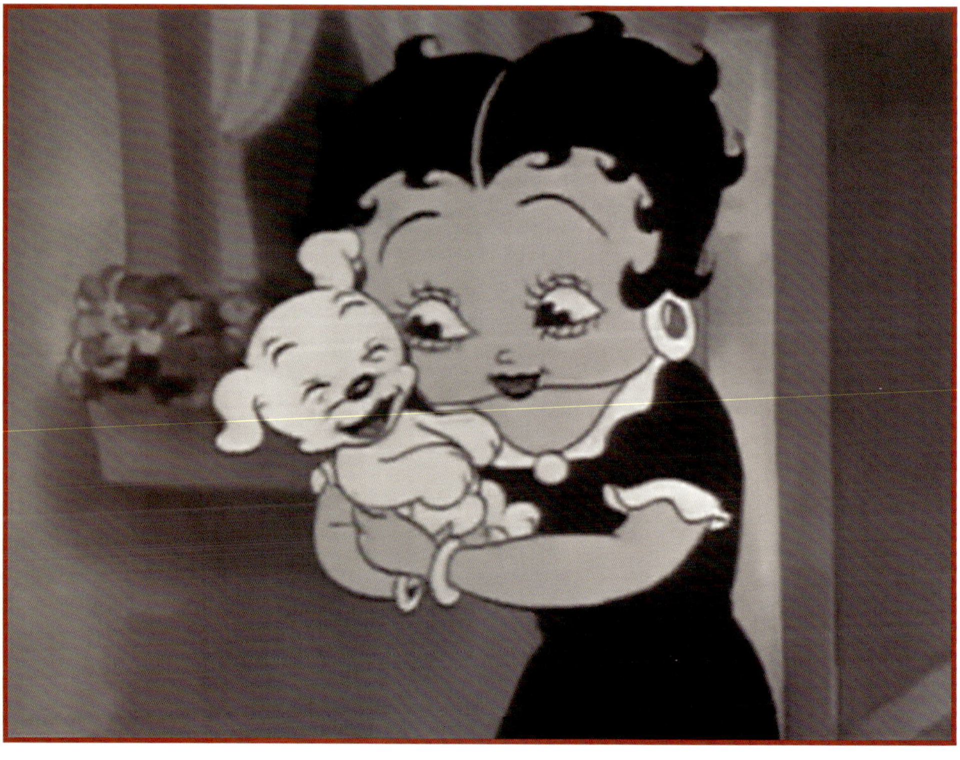

Women Today Enjoy Equality

True, it's not always a given and there are times when we have to remind the world of that equality. And, the phrase Betty uttered in 1932 when she said, "I can do anything a man can do," is accepted as a commonplace truth in today's world.

Women's Equality today is not just a dream anymore. It's a *fact*—a *reality*—supported by laws and regulations that guarantee equal opportunity and protection. Employers can no longer discriminate against women based on sex. And, if they do, we have legal recourse to help. This was unheard of when women faced regular discrimination in historical times. Woo-hoo!

Women Today Can Be Whomever They Want

Betty has always done exactly as she pleased. In an age when women often were relegated to domestic work as homemakers, mothers, and wives, Betty was a judge, a secretary, a train conductor, and a lion tamer. And, it's this spirit and sense of ability and promise that defines the modern woman.

Women Today Are Happier

Our awareness of the world around us has increased as has our ability to participate in it. We're more productive. Medical advances have enhanced our wellness and longevity. Technology has made our everyday lives easier. And, our computers and smartphones give us access to vast fields of knowledge, education, and information.

Women Today Wield Power

We are no longer referred to as the "fair" sex or the "weaker" sex. As a group, we finally are being recognized for our talent, contributions, and accomplishments.

We live with *passion, power*, and *purpose*. We have more *freedom* to express ourselves. And, with this freedom comes an *independence* that shines through everything we strive for and every dream we hold dear. Our predecessors would be *so proud* of us all!

We empower ourselves and empower each other. We decide what's best for us. And, we often run our race to independence solo—much like Betty always has. After all, Betty is the only female animated character in the world who has never been in a permanent relationship with a significant other. And, she does just great!

THE PRINCIPLE– Celebrate Your Singleness

Betty's Inspiration: Being single doesn't mean being alone.

Be Your Own New Best Friend. Do "me" things. Get out by yourself. Begin writing a journal. Take up a new hobby. Binge your favorite TV shows. Stay up late. Have pizza for breakfast. Enjoy being with yourself. This time is all about you!

Cultivate Your Sense of Self. Take this time to develop a stronger sense of who you are. Assess your talents, skills, and abilities. Figure out what you like about yourself and what you would like to improve. Now's the time for introspection and reflection.

Take Charge of Your Finances. The only finances with which you probably need to be concerned are your own. So, determine how you want to use your money. Prepare a budget. Decide how much you want to spend and how much you want to save. Set aside an amount each month to pay debts and open a long-term savings plan like an IRA or a 401K. This is a great habit that will serve you well all your life.

Enjoy Your Freedom. With few other responsibilities and no one to answer to, work hard at school or at your career. Travel. Focus on new projects and hobbies. Pamper yourself. Your time is your own!

Foster Other Relationships. Being single gives you more time to create and maintain new friendships. Have a girls' night out every week. Host a party. Plan activities that involve coworkers. Spend time with your family members. There is no significant other competing for your attention. You decide who you want to be with and when.

All in all, it's pretty darn amazing to be a modern woman in today's world. And, perhaps, if we asked Betty what her secret is to lasting relevance and Independence, she just might say,

"THE ABILITY TO ADAPT TO A CHANGING WORLD."

After all, every living creature must evolve in order to survive. And, no one demonstrates this better than Betty!

From her first appearance in 1930, she has changed with the times. A true chameleon, Betty's face and figure have changed. Her personal style and clothes have changed. Her interests, occupations, goals, and social causes have changed. Like the modern woman, over time she has become better—a *better version of herself*—changing on the outside while remaining true and steadfast on the inside.

Things that no longer serve well she has left in the past—while things that allow her to grow and evolve, she's grabbed with gusto. And, as we tackle the challenges of the twenty-first century, Betty remains a timeless symbol of feminine Strength, Power, Determination, and Independence.

And whatever Betty does, she always does it on her own terms. She continues to lend her hand and remain an Inspiration to all—forever *Embracing her Independence*.

"THE QUESTION ISN'T WHO IS GOING TO LET ME, IT'S WHO IS GOING TO STOP ME?"
—AYN RAND, PHILOSOPHER AND NOVELIST

DID YOU KNOW?

Betty Boop fans are called "Boopaholics."

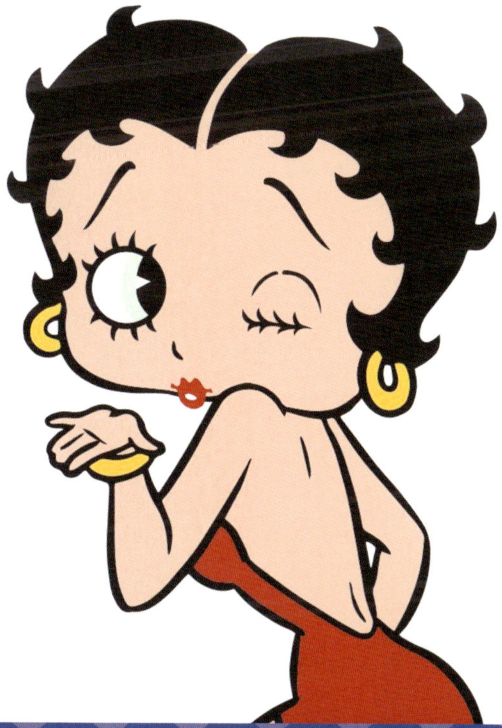

"STRONG WOMEN LIFT EACH OTHER UP!"

Chapter 2

Love Is All You Need

If there is one character that inspires people to think of love, kisses, and hearts, it's Betty Boop. From her signature red dress to her sweetheart personality to the hearts that seem to find their way into so much of her current imagery, Betty personifies love in everything she does.

Love is a common underlying theme throughout most of Betty's cartoons and messaging. Loving, wanting to be loved, or treating others with love were regular themes in Betty's original cartoons, which have the unique ability to not only entertain us, but to inspire us to think about love in all its forms, from relationships with animals to love for the people and things that surround us.

In a sense, through her many adventures, Betty teaches us that there are unlimited forms of love, and that we can rely on love to create a foundation for happiness, good relationships, compassion, and passionate living. When we expand our ideas of what exactly love is and the many places from which it can be given or received, we can experience love in our lives on entirely new levels.

Appropriately, Betty's very beginning was as a love interest for another popular Fleischer Studios character Bimbo in the 1930 cartoon *Dizzy Dishes*. However, her life has never been centered on romantic relationships. Instead, Betty embraces and thrives from love in all areas of her life, from her love for friends and family to her loyal dog companion Pudgy to her love of animals and helping others. She demonstrates that our hearts have limitless capacity for love, and how important it is to our vitality to welcome it in all of its manifestations.

> "MY FRIENDS ARE MY ESTATE."
> –EMILY DICKINSON, POET

When we shift our definition of love and allow it to encompass so much more than the traditional definition, we see that it is limitless. For some of us, like Betty, one of the greatest sources of love in our lives might simply be our circle of close friends whom over the years have become like family. And, the love of our life might just be our BFF or even a loving pet!

I WANNA BE LOVED BY YOU

Betty's version of the famous song "I Wanna Be Loved by You" was so loved by audiences that she became strongly associated with the hit, although it was actually written years earlier in 1928 by two gentleman named Herbert Stothart and Harry Ruby for a musical called *Good Boy.* Is there any tune that more clearly showcases our desire to be loved by another? Its relatable message of love, desire, and longing makes lyrics of the song so timeless.

I wanna be loved by you
Just you, and nobody else but you
I wanna be loved by you alone!
Boop-Oop-a-Doop!
I wanna be kissed by you
Just you, nobody else but you
I wanna be kissed by you alone!
I couldn't aspire
To anything higher
Than to feel the desire
To make you my own!
Boop-Oop-a-Doop!

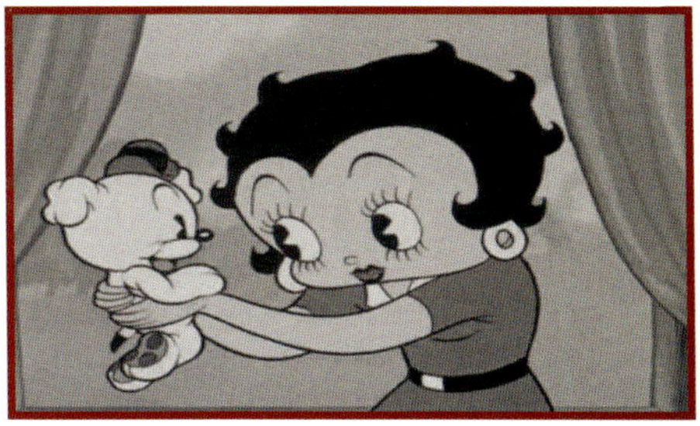

While Betty's version of the song may be one of the most widely known (although Marilyn Monroe's famous cover of the song in the 1959 film *Some Like It Hot* is right up there as well), the beloved tune has actually been performed over the decades by a wide variety of famous artists, including Jack Lemmon, Tina Louise, Barry Manilow (in a duet with the Marilyn Monroe version), and even Sinéad O'Connor.

The famous song is just one of many examples of how Betty has personified love throughout the years. There are so many great lessons and messages about love that can be drawn from Betty and her adventures, we thought we would share a few highlights with you. Here are four key elements about love that can inspire the expansion of love in our lives, as well as change the way we see love.

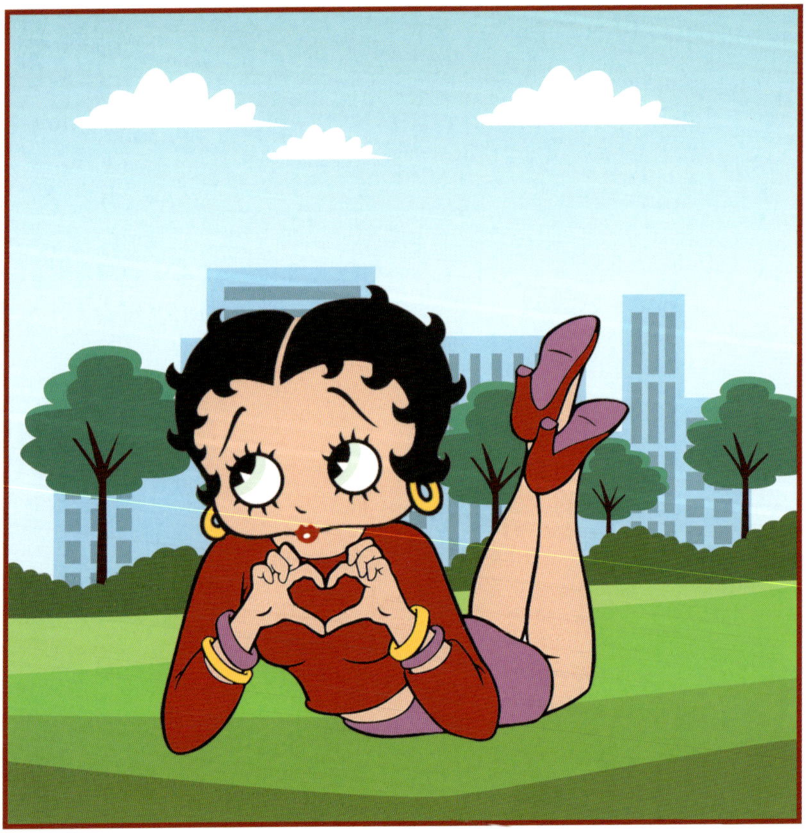

THE PRINCIPLE–
Betty's Lessons on Love

Betty's Inspiration: Love is always available no matter where you are.

Know That Love Comes in Many Forms. When we think of the word "love," most of us tend to first think of romantic love. But our love for animals, a stunning sunset, or a beautiful garden also can bring us great joy. The variety of love sources is endless and Betty shows us countless examples of this throughout her cartoons and messaging. It's all about expanding our view of love and learning to recognize the many great places from which we can give and receive love.

Try a Little Love Experiment. Take a piece of paper and write down all the people, places, and things in your life that bring you a little (or big!) spark of love. Anything that comes to mind counts—there are no rules! Pets, family, a favorite city, self-love, love you feel from a favorite robe that has kept you warm on countless nights . . . nothing is insignificant. When you do this, you may feel a bit surprised (and happy!) when you see just how much love is actually in your life!

Love for Nature and for Life. There is something very special about the deep love we can all feel for—and from—nature and life itself when we allow it in. The deep connection we can experience when surrounded by blue skies, trees, soaring birds, mountains, and water is a very unique love. It reminds us how beautiful life can be, even through the hard times. Next time you're feeling the need for a dose of powerful love, step outside or go somewhere beautiful such as a local park and really allow yourself to soak in what's around you. You'll feel energized and centered.

Love for Complete Strangers. Have you ever been relaxing at a park or walking through a shopping center and received an instant blast of love when you witness a family playing in a fountain or a daddy picking up and swinging around his little girl? Isn't that a fun and wonderful feeling? Getting out of the house and going for a stroll in places where people gather for happy reasons such as family time, shopping, or entertainment can be great for the soul! The love you can give and experience energetically with others without even exchanging words is a beautiful thing.

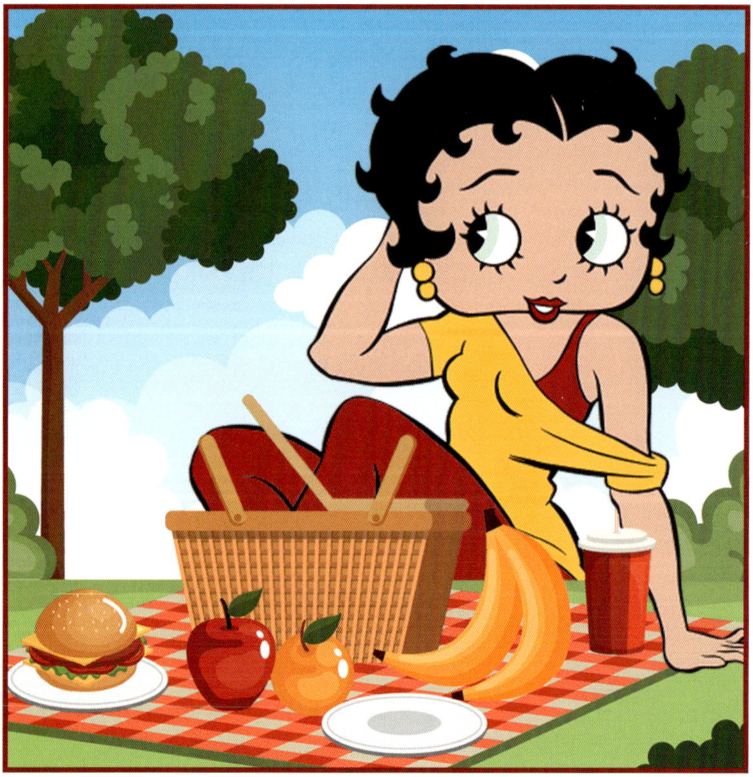

LOVE FOR OUR ANIMAL FRIENDS

In the sweet cartoon *Betty Boop with Henry, the Funniest Living American*, a young boy Henry falls in love with a puppy at Betty's pet store, but doesn't have enough money to adopt him. Betty, touched by Henry's love for the pup, decides to let Henry work at the store so he can earn the puppy. She happily sings, "Everybody oughta have a pet!"

Betty's advice is even backed by science! Numerous studies have shown that pets are good for our health and can add joy to our lives. Pets can reduce depression, anxiety, loneliness, and help keep us active. They can also help us live longer! A 2017 study in Sweden followed 3.4 million men and women between the ages of forty and eighty and tracked their health records for approximately twelve years. The study concluded that for people who live alone, owning a dog significantly reduced risk of cardiovascular related deaths by up to 36 percent as well as overall causes of death by up to 33 percent. Who knew loving our pets could be so healthy?

Love for animals of course can extend beyond our pets to all animals. You don't need to have a pet to enjoy animals and the joy they can bring. From sitting outside watching birds and other wildlife to visiting your local zoo, there are countless ways to enjoy the pure, innocent love that comes from our connection to all the world's creatures.

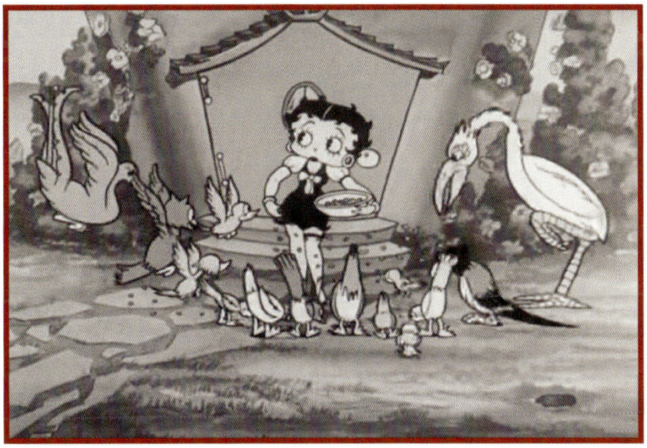

Betty's love for animals is an element in many of her original cartoons and comes through clear as day. She has animal friends of all kinds. We also know that Betty's most loyal companion is her pup, Pudgy. He goes with her practically everywhere. He's definitely a great source of love in Betty's life. It's very clear she was on to something long before there were studies to prove it.

ALL GOOD THINGS BEGIN WITH SELF-LOVE

When we can truly love and accept ourselves, life is brighter, more joyful, and definitely more fun! All of Betty's actions begin with love, and many are based on self-love. From the way she stands up for herself in challenging situations to the way she is always seeking adventures, Betty is determined to live her dreams and have fun doing it. She has boundaries, takes breaks, and makes time for things she's passionate about, which are all acts of self-love.

Betty even teaches others the importance of self-love. In her classic cartoon *You're Not Built That Way*, Betty tries to teach Pudgy the importance of accepting himself just the way he is when she spots him trying to change himself to be more like a bigger, stronger dog. In the end, Pudgy learns a valuable lesson and is happier for it.

So why is self-love so hard for many of us? And how can we get better about it? Well, first we can remember that we should be extending to ourselves all the love that we so willingly and openly give to others. Our hearts have a limitless capacity for love, and when we treat ourselves with love and kindness, it supports our ability to show even more love toward others in our lives.

Second, try making self-care the number one item on your list. You'll often see images of Betty relaxing at the beach, walking in the park, enjoying a spa day, reading a book, or tending to the flowers in her garden. She takes time for herself! This is definitely linked to why she is so joyful and full of positivity. Betty knows how to put her needs first, and this allows her to share her very best self with everyone in her life.

Finally, we can remember that we are all our own very best friend and then begin to treat ourselves that way. We would never say anything negative or be mean to our dearest friends, so why do we do this to ourselves? Betty Boop is her own BFF, and works hard to be a loving friend to herself. This is something we can all practice.

> "LOVE YOURSELF FIRST AND EVERYTHING ELSE FALLS INTO LINE."
> —LUCILLE BALL, ACTRESS AND COMEDIAN

Try creating a list of small shifts you can make to be more loving toward yourself. Do you need to clear some things from your calendar so you have more time for yourself? Do you need to adjust your schedule a bit so you can get more sleep? Would it be helpful to your overall health and energy to make some small positive changes to your diet and drink more water? Small changes can create big results and are very doable.

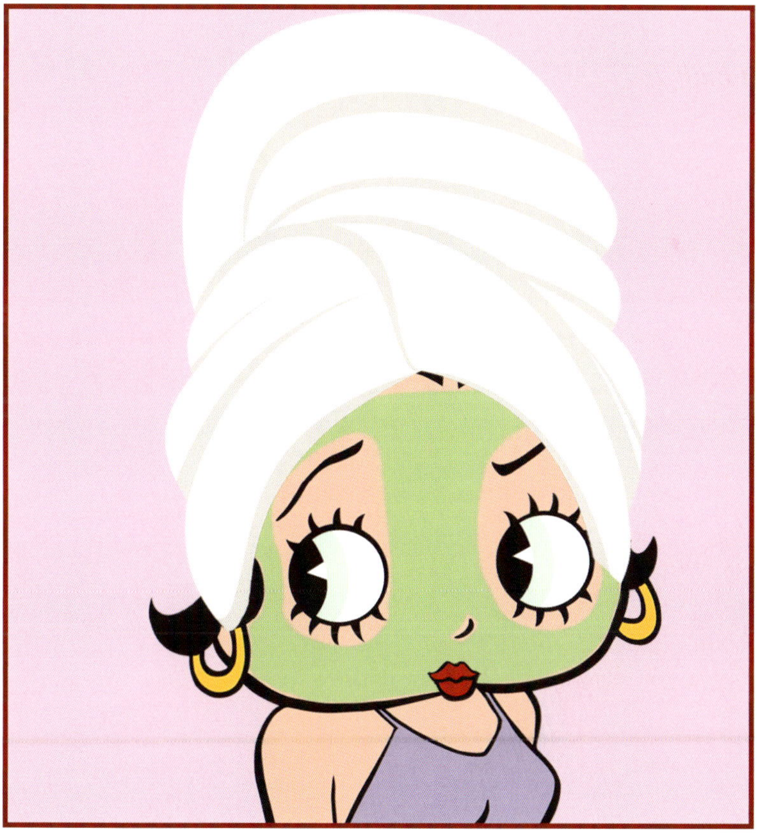

THE PRINCIPLE–
Celebrate Love

Betty's Inspiration: When love is the primary driving force, you can never go wrong.

Let Love Motivate You. By allowing love to be your driving force, it can make even the most overwhelming of endeavors flow with joy and ease. This is especially helpful when a task ahead seems tedious. When you tap into the love behind why you're doing something and the feeling you'll have when you're finished doing it, it can make even the most daunting of tasks seem much more doable. When you feel unmotivated by something, close your eyes and think about what form of love is behind your want or need to do that particular thing. Love is fantastic inspiration!

Trust in Love. When we've been hurt or heartbroken in some way, it can sometimes be a challenge to trust in love again. It's important to remember that it's not actually the *love* that caused the hurt, but that one specific situation, which is separate from the love. Love itself does not hurt, and when we understand this, it becomes easier to trust in love. Another thought to ponder: sometimes hurt or grief is a sign that you have loved well! And, although it can be bittersweet, loving well is something to be celebrated and repeated.

Know That Love Is Limitless. You have infinite kinds of love within you to serve as inspiration and foundation building blocks for almost anything you might do. All you need to do is tap into it and let it flow, just like Max did when creating his characters and films. Whether it's love for a person you're going to see or doing something for, or love for an occupation, place, or hobby—let it be noticeably present by deliberately focusing on it and then allowing it to support and motivate you.

RE-THINK ROMANCE

When we think of love, often we also think of romance. And, when we think of romance, most of us first think of a candlelight dinner or roses from a special someone, but there's an entirely different way to see it (outside of love relationships) that can invite abundant romance into your life from many difference places! Romance can be found and enjoyed almost everywhere if you're open to seeing it—no partner required (this is a secret Betty knows for sure!).

Romance can be found in the spring wildflowers, the ocean, the rain, and the stars. It's in the care that you put into cooking yourself a meal or shopping for your favorite groceries. It's in a quiet evening at home watching a favorite TV show. It's in decorating a home, clean sheets, hot bubble baths, travel, and friendships. Life is full of romance! Isn't that wonderful?

Betty Boop knows how to find the romance in many different situations. You might find her swooning over a flower or noticing the beauty in a seemingly ordinary day. Finding romance in everyday situations and things is a practice that can be developed, and once you become pretty good at it (which you will!), life becomes that much more delicious!

Begin looking for romance in all the parts of your everyday life and soon you'll be enjoying your days with a completely different view. All it takes is a small shift in perspective and suddenly so many things around you can evoke swoon-worthy feelings! Isn't just the notion itself romantic?

DO ALL THINGS WITH LOVE

Here's another little secret about love. It's a wonderful foundation for *any* intention. In fact, it should be the foundation for *all* your intentions when you get right down to it. When you approach life and everything you do with love as your motivation, it makes everything sweeter and more purposeful. And, as we mentioned in our last tip section, it makes even the most daunting tasks seem more doable and joyful. Just think of the positive energy this approach can cultivate!

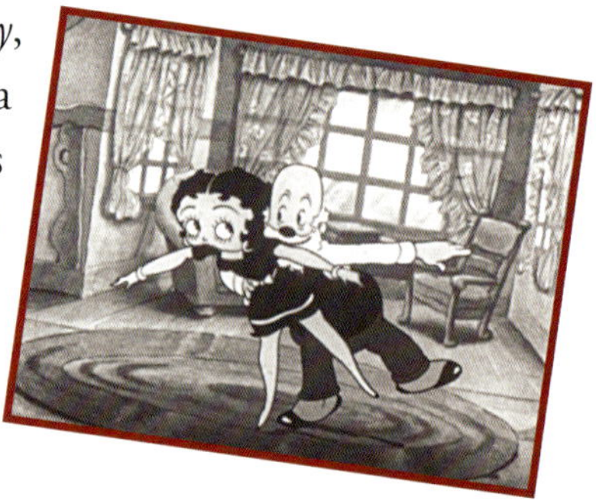

In the classic cartoon *Betty Boop and Grampy*, Betty Boop is on her way to Grampy's house for a celebration and is so excited about going, she invites several friends she meets along the way to come and share in the fun. Betty's intention of spreading joy and love, as well as showing Grampy how much she appreciates his hospitality, results in a great time for all. It's clear that Betty's love for all things Grampy, and even in her catchy song-and-dance approach to walking over to his house (seriously—watch this cartoon and you'll be singing her little tune about Grampy's house all day), is the foundation that helped to create a successful party.

I'm on my way to Grampy's house
Where he always treats me nice
Always something on the ice
Over at Grampy's house!

Betty herself was a complete labor of love for her creator, Max Fleischer. In the classic cartoon *Betty Boop's Rise to Fame*, both animation and live action are combined when Max is being interviewed by a newspaper reporter and is explaining the process of producing Betty Boop's cartoons. As Max lovingly draws Betty on a sketchpad, an animated Betty suddenly springs to life and actually jumps off the paper to join both Max and the reporter in the film! It clearly was that love Max had for art, animation, and his characters that became the foundation of Betty, her loving character, and her years of success.

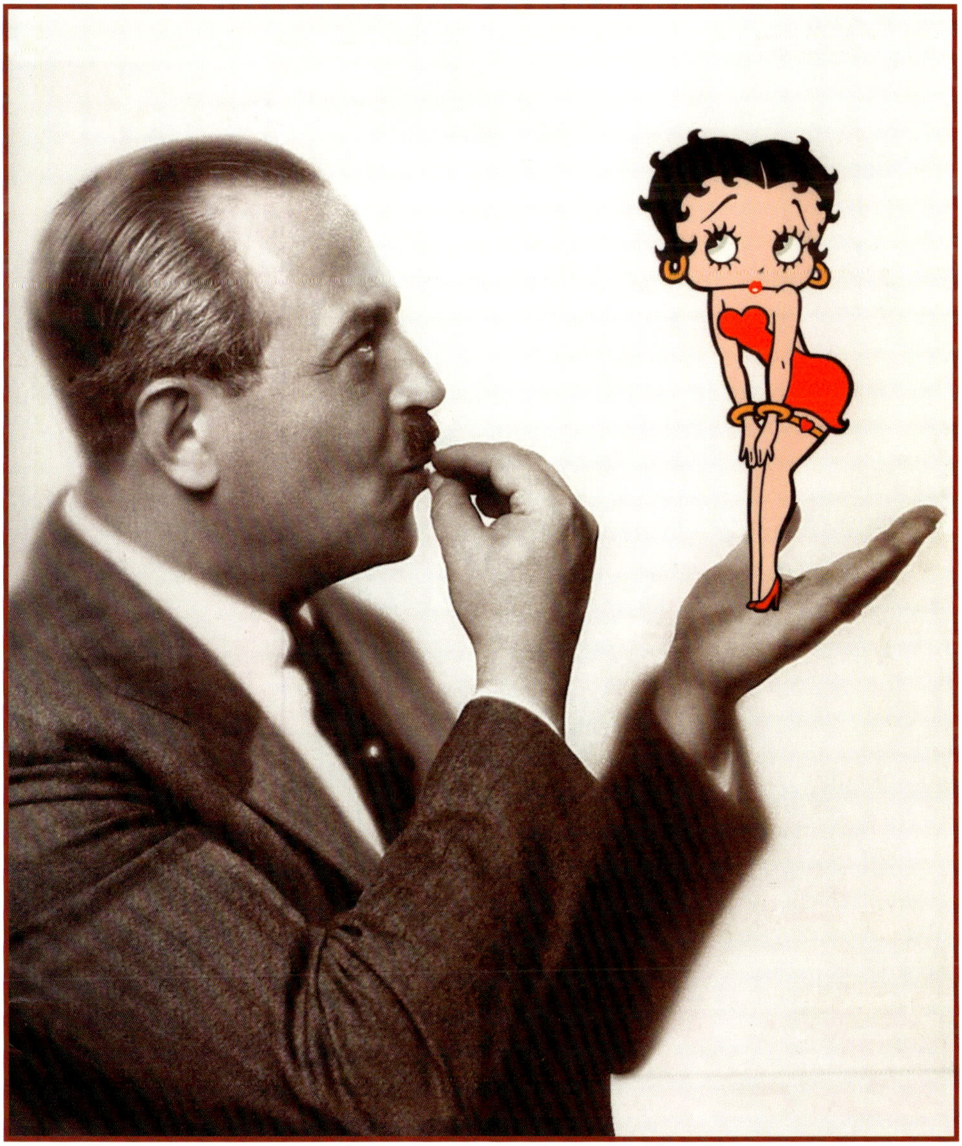

"LOVE IS THE SUBSTANCE OF ALL LIFE. EVERYTHING IS CONNECTED IN LOVE. ABSOLUTELY EVERYTHING."
—JULIA CAMERON, TEACHER AND AUTHOR

LOVE AS A TOP PRIORITY

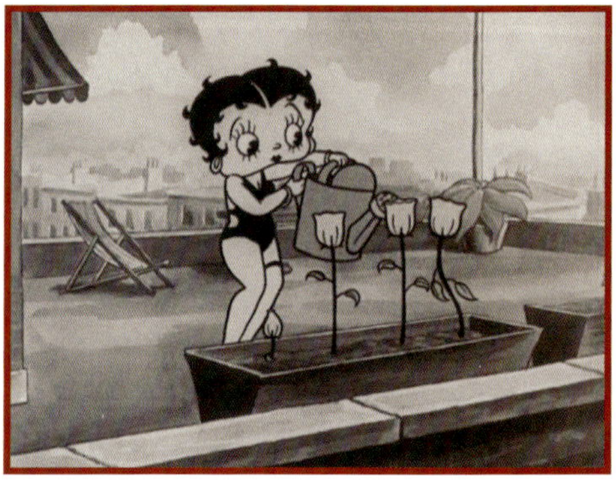

With the busyness of everyday life, it's so easy to fall into the trap of neglecting love and taking it for granted. Love, like a garden, needs to be watered and tended in order to flourish. Can you think of times in your life when you put other things ahead of love? Where there may have even been consequences?

One of the most important rules to live by is to always practice placing all the forms of love in your life at the top of your priority list. Making the people, places, and things that you love a top priority (including yourself!) is a sure way to help keep all areas of your life happy and thriving. It's also important to incorporate love in your daily interactions as well as remembering that, in some way, love is the motive behind all you do.

CULTIVATING LOVE

When it comes to prioritizing love, we must pay special attention to our relationships. Science has shown that nurturing relationships and cultivating love can help you be happier, healthier, and more successful in your life overall.

There are many studies that show how important it is to care for our relationships. Perhaps the most fascinating is Harvard's Grant and Glueck study.

For more than seventy-five years, researchers tracked the emotional health and well-being of two groups of men! Yes, seventy-five years! How incredible is that? The Grant study tracked 436 men growing up in the inner-city Boston area from 1937 to 2014, and the Glueck study tracked 239 male graduates from Harvard's classes of 1939 to 1944. In the end, the Director of the Harvard Study of Adult Development said, "The clearest message that we get from this 75-year study is this: Good relationships keep us happier and healthier. Period."

This is great news! It's great news because it confirms that when we shift our priorities to put love at the top (over money, career, success) we're truly empowering ourselves to live our very best lives.

GRATITUDE AS A FORM OF LOVE

Another way to see love is in the forms of gratitude and grace. Each is actually a form of love, and when viewed this way, can greatly expand the love we recognize and feel in our lives. When we give gratitude to someone else, or to the world for something in our life, it's actually an expression of love. Gratitude has the power to return us from any place of negativity and returns us to a place of love. It also can help us to love more unconditionally by removing any judgmental thoughts and replacing them with love. When we're grateful to someone, there is no room for judgment or resentment. So, it's safe to say that practicing gratitude is part of cultivating love.

PRACTICING GRATITUDE

Gratitude is truly a practice. And, when we practice it enough, it becomes a wonderful habit. A great way to begin is by simply taking a minute or two each morning before you get out of bed to reflect on what you're grateful for. You also can close your eyes and do this any time you feel like you may be losing sight of all that you *do* have (rather than focusing on all you wish you had). It's a great little habit to adopt!

When you have a conflict with someone you value in your life, try closing your eyes and thinking about what you are thankful for in that person. You'll see how quickly the conflict feels softer, and you may even see a new path to resolving the conflict that had escaped you before.

When you're feeling drained or down, try making a list of everything you're grateful for in your life and you'll find yourself uplifted every single time. Gratitude is a fantastic spirit lifter! With practice, you'll find yourself turning to gratitude as a go-to state of mind in a wide assortment of life's situations.

GRACE IN LOVE

When we notice the grace that is all around us in our lives at all times, we are really noticing love. When we train ourselves to notice the love all around, to focus on gratitude, and to look for the good in everything we can, we are living in grace. Living in grace, like cultivating gratitude, takes practice.

Living in grace means developing a deep knowing within that you are always loved and supported, by those you love, by life, and by any spiritual practice you may choose to embrace in your life. Love and support are always there, and a strong trust of this is a key element in our emotional well-being. It's even in the smallest of things, such as happy coincidences that work in your favor or a beautiful day when you really feel like you need sunshine. Learning to *see* the grace is the foundation for living it.

Allowing gratitude and grace to fill your heart as often as possible can greatly expand the overall presence of love in our lives, as well as bring greater joy and peace.

THE ART OF FORGIVENESS

Forgiveness in many ways is actually a form of love. It's love extended toward another who has wronged you or made a mistake. It's love extended toward yourself when you forgive *you*. Perhaps most importantly, it's a form of self-love because when you choose to forgive, you are freeing yourself from holding on to the daunting weight of resentment and negativity.

Let's chat about practicing self-forgiveness. Being willing to forgive our own mistakes (everyone makes them—even Betty!) and accept ourselves just as we are is a great foundation for self-love, and the freedom that comes from it is key to living our best life. Part of self-forgiveness is knowing that you did the best you could in that moment with the knowledge or energy you had at the time, and in the emotional place you were in at the time.

Mistakes have a purpose. They're part of how we learn, grow, and become stronger. So, work hard to be sure you're forgiving yourself for absolutely everything. Send love to the version of yourself that made that mistake, let go, and move forward as a wiser person.

"FORGIVE YOURSELF. FORGIVE YOUR CELLS, YOUR BONES, YOUR TISSUES. FORGIVE YOUR THOUGHTS AND ACTIONS. FORGIVE IT ALL."
—KRIS CARR, AUTHOR AND WELLNESS ADVOCATE

Forgiving others also is a form of self-love, as it frees you from resentment and negative energy. It prevents events of the past from crippling us in the present. It allows us to be free from heavy emotional baggage so we can live our life in a more productive and positive way.

To be clear, forgiving someone does not mean forgetting what has occurred. You can forgive someone while remembering their wrongful actions and the hurt they may have caused you. Remembering allows us to learn and grow from a negative or painful experience. This is how we become stronger, wiser, and more capable.

And most important of all, we need to learn how to forgive without expecting—or receiving—an apology. People don't always apologize for their mistakes or for hurting others (and some are actually *not* sorry). Remember that the act of forgiving is for *you*, not for them.

There will always be people who hurt, attack, or betray us. Shocking and surprising behavior in people is part and parcel of the human condition and will always be present in our life. But the great news here is that we can choose how we respond to it and refuse to allow pain and negativity to overshadow who we are and the joy we feel. Forgiveness is the key to lightness, freedom of the soul, and living fully in the moment.

LOVE'S POWERFUL FORCE

Love is possibly the most powerful force in the universe. It has the power to heal, to bring people together, and to transform lives. It has the power to inspire greater generosity, kindness, and compassion. When we choose to live and see the world through loving eyes, in a way, we actually become love.

Give yourself the gift of living in and embracing love from all of its sources. You'll be amazed at the new levels of joy and peace this will bring to your heart.

DID YOU KNOW?

Betty Boop's beloved pup Pudgy first appeared in the 1934 animated film *Betty Boop's Little Pal.*

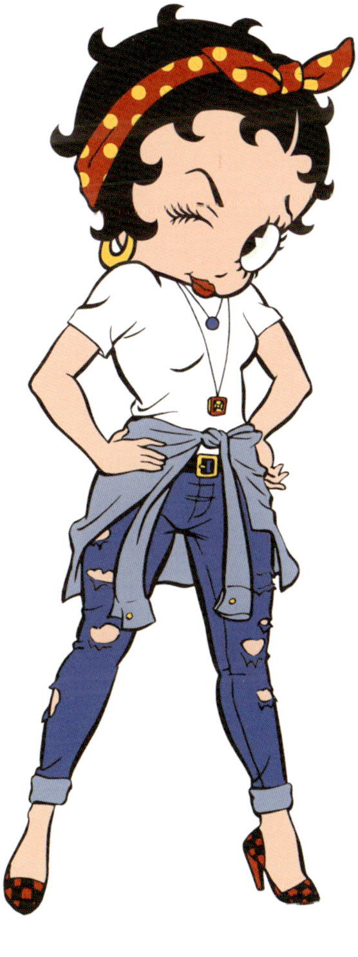

"DO ALL THINGS WITH LOVE!"

CHAPTER 3

A Little Kindness Goes a Long Way

Kindness is one of the most powerful forces in the world. It can resolve conflict, touch our hearts, and make us feel seen and heard. Like love, kindness was a theme in many of Betty's original cartoons, and it's a message she still shares today.

With daily exposure to negative news, Internet trolls, stress-inducing political chatter, and overall digital overwhelm, we're in dire need of a new focus on kindness as a foundation for all we do. The only way to combat the unkindness in the world is to cultivate more authentic, loving kindness. This can be done in a number of ways, from small acts like warm smiles and friendly hellos to volunteering for a charitable cause that's important to you. Simple acts of kindness (both given and received) can make every day feel lighter, more energetic, and better overall.

Several of Betty's early cartoons demonstrate the importance of kindness and compassion in powerful ways that are still so relevant and current in today's world.

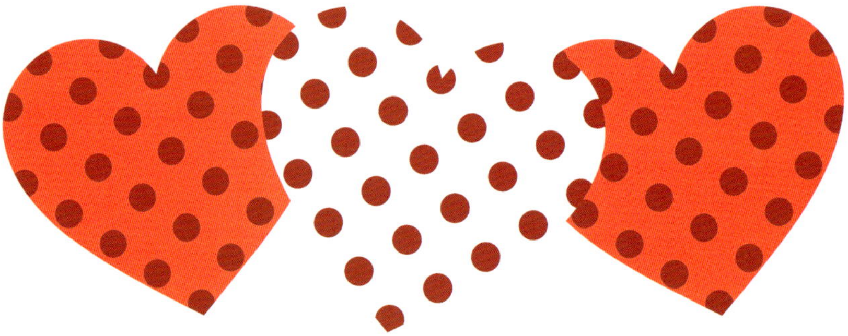

In *A Song a Day*, Betty takes care of injured animals, singing about how a little kindness can make life worth living:

An understanding touch, a sympathetic word
can drive away those troubles like the song of a bird.

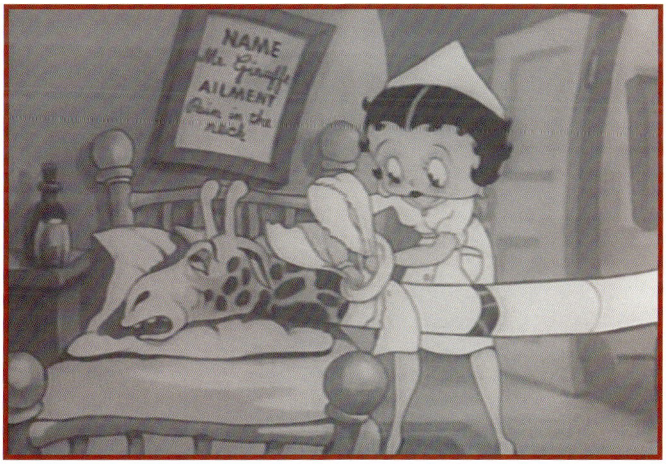

KINDNESS AS A SUPERPOWER

What's great about kindness is that it really begins with the simplest of thoughts and acts. As Betty says, "*an understanding touch, a sympathetic word* . . ." can make all the difference. And, on the surface, kindness seems like such a simple concept. But, the truth is that it's an extraordinarily powerful force and there are many layers in play to consider. With a deeper understanding and with dedicated practice, kindness can actually become a superpower!

So, what does it take to make kindness one of your superpowers? Here are six elements to consider when looking to expand the superpower of kindness in your life. Just think of the healing and joy that would occur in the world if everyone stepped up their kindness game. Are you ready?

Kindness Takes Practice

Most of the elements we cover in this book can be thought of as skills that can be practiced, expanded, and sharpened. Kindness is no different. Of course, most people are kind in their thoughts and hearts, but not everyone practices it as frequently as they would like. Being more deliberate about acts of kindness can help create more of a natural habit out of it, and therefore can increase the positive effects of it in our lives and the lives of those around us. It is teachable, and we can teach ourselves as well through practice. Kindness creates—and attracts—more kindness.

So where do we begin in practicing more kindness? The good news here is that the best place to start is with small goals, such as, "I will go out of my way to do something kind for someone else three times today." Then, be sure to deliberately perform those acts. They don't have to be big or inconvenient. A heartfelt email telling someone you appreciate them, complimenting and thanking the check-out clerk at the grocery store, or a small contribution to a charity drive a friend is running are all achievable and spread goodness. Starting with doable goals like this (and then expanding from there) is a great way to begin creating new habits out of kindness. You'll not only make others smile and feel good, you'll feel great too!

Kindness Is Healthy

Numerous studies have shown that kindness can improve our health and overall well-being. It's even been shown that simply witnessing acts of kindness can increase the good chemical oxytocin in our brain, which can reduce stress, blood pressure, and help with overall heart health.

Acts of kindness can even increase your energy! So, if you're feeling sluggish this could be a great way to gain some increased zing in your step. In one study at the University of California–Berkeley's Greater Good Science Center showed that nearly 50 percent of people feel greater strength and increased energy after helping others. Many others in the study reported feeling greater self-esteem and feelings of calmness. Who doesn't want all that?

Research also has shown that kinder people live longer, healthier lives across the board. So, the old saying "When you give, you get" is actually very true on many levels. Now, of course, these facts are not the primary motivation for being giving and kind, but they're definitely a huge bonus!

People Remember Kindness

The great poet and author Maya Angelou once said, "I've learned that people will forget what you said, people will forget what you did, but people will never forget how you made them feel." This is absolutely true. And, the way people feel after they experience kindness is an unforgettable positive feeling that lasts long after the actual event.

Can you recall a time in your life when someone offered you an incredible act of kindness? When you think about it, it likely brings up all those warm and positive feelings that you felt right after it happened. You probably remember that person very fondly. If someone asked you to describe that person, kind would likely be one of the first things you mention.

Many who have watched a number of Betty's classic cartoons might mention kindness as one of her many positive qualities if asked to describe her. They may or may not remember specific things she did, but the energy of her frequent kind acts and compassionate outlook sticks in the mind.

Each one of us would undoubtedly like to be remembered in a positive way by people we meet, and spreading kindness is the best path to help make that happen. Of course, true kindness comes from the heart without expectation of anything in return, but isn't it great that there are all these bonuses?

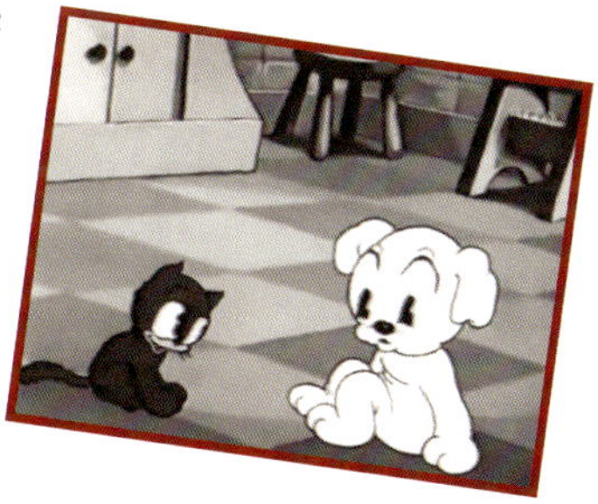

Kindness Isn't Always Easy

One of the biggest things to understand about kindness is that it takes effort, and sometimes it takes sacrifice. Kindness and selflessness really do go hand in hand.

In the 1938 cartoon *Pudgy and the Lost Kitten*, Betty's adorable sidekick Pudgy comes across a little lost kitten and brings him home to Betty. Both Betty and Pudgy give up their day to help the lost little one, feeding, bathing, and looking for its mother.

The lost kitten ordeal ends up being a big pain in the you-know-what for Pudgy! The kitten eats most of Pudgy's food, plays with his tail (sticking it with sharp kitten claws!), and tries to take over his bed. But, Pudgy puts up with it all, and even goes out looking for the kitten's mom. He finally finds her frantically looking for her baby, and brings them back together. Needless to say, Pudgy is thrilled when the kitten is out of his life, but Betty still cuddles him and tells him how wonderful he is for helping the little guy.

Be Kind to You

This one can sometimes be the most challenging. Like self-love, sometimes the last person we extend our kindness to is our own self. But the truth is, we owe ourselves the kindness that we try so hard to freely give others!

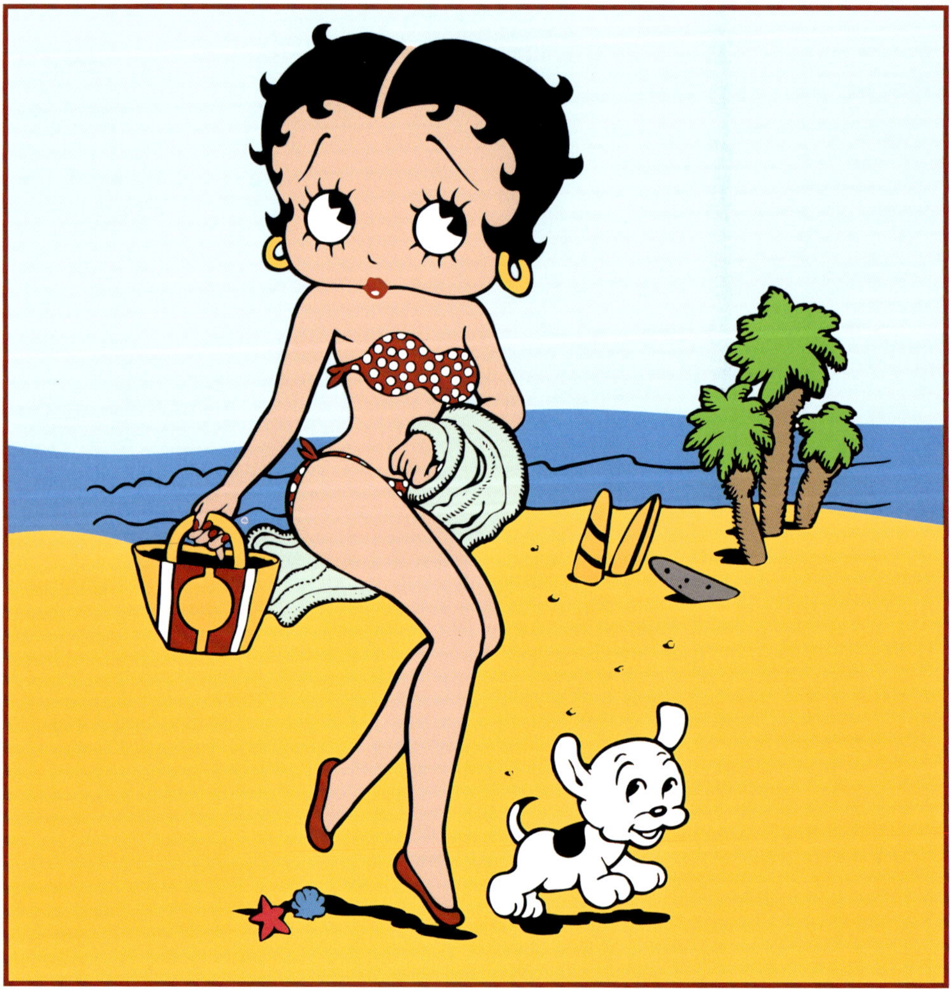

When life gets busy, it's so easy to neglect our own needs, be hard on ourselves when we're already feeling overwhelmed, and even say unkind things about ourselves that we would never even think to say about someone else. It's so important to remember that the person in your life most deserving of your own kindness and generosity is *you*.

As we mentioned in the last section, kindness takes deliberate effort and it isn't always easy. This is especially true when it comes to being kind to ourselves. When the day has been long and stressful, and you feel like you've got a zillion things on your plate, it's so easy to put everyone else first. This is when we most need to consider being extra gentle, kind, and easy on ourselves.

We cannot force ourselves out of a difficult emotional place before we're ready to heal, or bully ourselves out of bad habits we know we need to change. Be patient with yourself and give yourself the space, time, love, and support to go through things in your own time and in your own way. Remember that your soul is always deserving of your kindness, and never apologize for doing what you need to do to be kind to yourself and protect your peace.

It's also important to take time to *play*. Allowing time in your schedule to take breaks, take time to reflect, and do fun things that you enjoy is all part of self-care, but also is a tremendous act of kindness toward yourself. Don't forget to allow time for fun!

One more important thing to consider: Being kind to yourself includes purposefully surrounding yourself with people who are *kind to you*. We all have the choice of who to surround ourselves with and being highly aware of making sure the people in our lives are kind, loving souls

"NOBODY'S PERFECT, SO GIVE YOURSELF CREDIT FOR EVERYTHING YOU'RE DOING RIGHT, AND BE KIND TO YOURSELF WHEN YOU STRUGGLE."
—LORI DESCHENE, AUTHOR AND BLOGGER

who inspire in some way is a wonderful act of kindness to ourselves! Distance yourself from anyone who doesn't treat you with kindness and respect—another great practice for living your most bold and balanced life.

Those Who Are the Hardest to Be Kind to Are the Ones Who Need It Most

One of the most challenging elements of kindness is to remember that people who are difficult, negative, or otherwise not in our favor are likely those who need our kindness the most. It can be difficult at times to find it within ourselves to go out of our way to be kind to those we disagree with, who are unkind, or who are hard to love. Especially when those are generally the people that we'd like to distance ourselves from. But, the ability to be kind to unkind people is part of the true meaning of kindness without expectations. And, with a little creativity, we can still extend kindness while distancing ourselves at the same time.

When someone is rude, obnoxious, or does something we just don't agree with, it can be tempting to respond with harsh words or a cold shoulder. It's important to remember that more times than not, when someone lashes out or acts like a jerk it's because they're hurting inside in some way. Knowing this makes it a bit easier to respond with kindness. By being kind to a negative person, you have the power to change the entire situation. This is where the superpower of kindness can really come into play!

One of the last things a person who has been mean or negative is expecting is kindness from someone else. When we're kind to someone who is behaving this way, or to someone who has wronged us, many times you can feel the energy of the situation change right then or there. They are disarmed. The mood lightens. Their attitude and approach may change entirely. The old saying, "Kill them with kindness" is a powerful approach to any negative situation!

HOW TO OFFER KINDNESS TO A DIFFICULT PERSON

Offering kindness to people who are mean, negative, or difficult can require a great deal of strength and patience. Let's chat about just a few of the ways we can approach this challenge.

THE PRINCIPLE– Stretching Your Kindness Muscles

Betty's Inspiration: Everyone you meet is going through some kind of challenge. Be Kind.

Tap into Compassion. When you encounter a person who is unkind or who triggers you in some way, take a breath and try to think about what this person might be experiencing or feeling inside that's causing them to act this way. Anger? Frustration? Hurt? When you shift your perspective to understanding and compassion, it makes it much easier to feel that the mean person in question may actually deserve your kindness after all.

Self-Reflection Can Provide Great Insight. In addition to making an effort to more compassionately understand what's behind the actions of another person, a bit of self-understanding and reflection can help too. Sometimes we are triggered by a person due to something inside of us that has nothing to do with that particular person. Realizing that some negative feelings are *entirely* our own doing can be very enlightening and help to dissolve hard feelings.

Empathy Works Wonders. "I sense you're having a hard time." "I feel you're unhappy." Verbal support is a tonic. Reach out. Share an experience you have in common with someone who's hurting. Make someone feel welcome and included by extending an invitation or two. Catch another off guard with an unexpected act of kindness. It can result in miracles! And, it can certainly make life easier for all when working with stressed, disappointed, or grouchy coworkers and family members.

Know There Are Some People Who Will Not Respond in a Positive Way (and That's Okay). There are some people—no matter how nice you are—who will continue to be mean, negative, or refuse to receive help. *Be kind anyway.* They may come around, they may not, but you can never go wrong by adding kindness to the mix in any situation. We can't please everyone all the time.

It's also important to remember that some people may be in such a deeply painful or negative place that they're not ready to receive kindness—or they may not feel deserving. This doesn't mean that deep down they don't recognize or appreciate your effort, and it's very likely they'll remember it with gratitude when they're in a better place.

"KINDNESS IS ONE OF THE GREATEST GIFTS YOU CAN BESTOW UPON ANOTHER. IF SOMEONE IS IN NEED, LEND THEM A HELPING HAND. DO NOT WAIT FOR A THANK YOU. TRUE KINDNESS LIES WITHIN THE ACT OF GIVING WITHOUT THE EXPECTATION OF SOMETHING IN RETURN."

—KATHARINE HEPBURN, ACTRESS AND HUMANITARIAN

KINDNESS BEFORE OUR EYES

It may seem like there is a lot of unkindness and negativity in the world. However, when you look for it, kindness (like love) can be found in so many places! Looking for and recognizing kindness wherever it appears is a wonderful joy booster. Think about the warm and fuzzy feeling you get when you simply witness an act of kindness, whether on TV or in real life. You don't even have to be the giver or the receiver of the kindness to benefit!

Remembering that all kindness has a ripple effect and can bring good feelings and inspiration to those who simply witness it is another great motivator to make it a greater presence in your life. With this in mind, we thought it would be fun to point out a few of the more modern examples of kindness that are popping up in our world and spreading all kinds of goodness! These are just a few of the many creative ways people, schools, organizations, and companies from all over are working to share and inspire kindness.

Pop-Up Free Tiny Libraries

You may have seen them. Adorable wooden structures full of books popping up in front yards and on school campuses around the world—take a book, leave a book! It's free and fun and oozes kindness. Children and adults alike are taking part in the community book exchanges made possible by these sweet miniature libraries, which are inspiring more human connection in addition to encouraging more reading. There's even a non-profit organization called Little Free Library leading the way to helping people set up these tiny free libraries in their communities. Inspired? Visit them online to find out how to set one up in your community!

Social Media Fundraisers

If you're on social media, you've probably noticed an increase in charitable fundraising online, and even the tiniest donations are welcome! Social media companies have added features to their platforms to make it as easy as the click of a button to set up a fundraiser for your favorite charity and invite all your friends to contribute.

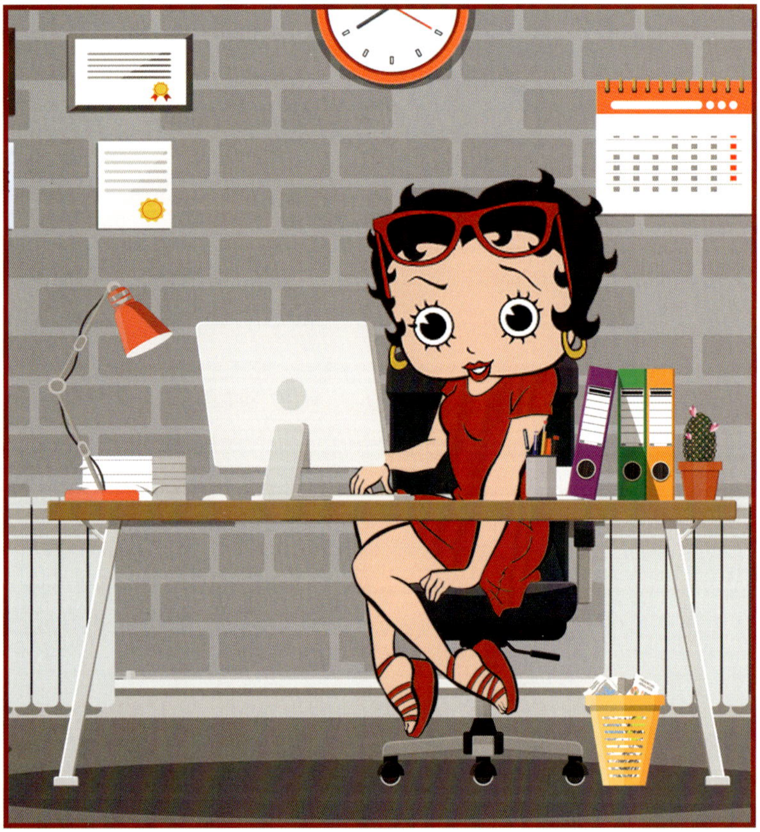

All this giving is expanding the energy of kindness across the Internet and inspiring tremendous generosity and goodwill. This is definitely one of the more positive things happening on social media today, and it's a great way for individuals to make a big impact through small donations. Clickable kindness!

Crowdfunding

When you think about the concept of crowdfunding—the financing of people's dreams via many small donations from a lot of different people who support their idea—it really does have kindness written all over it! Thousands of entrepreneurs and artists of all ages have raised the funds needed to launch their companies, projects, or inventions through online crowdfunding platforms. Not just from friends and family, but from total strangers who saw their idea online and wanted to help make it a reality. Talk about a great example of random acts of kindness!

Crowdfunding has even been used to help families raise needed funds to pay medical bills, and to help prospective students pay for higher education they couldn't otherwise afford. Crowdfunding is a wonderful example of the tremendous impact that many people coming together to extend small acts of kindness can have.

The above examples of kindness happening before our eyes in today's world are just a drop in the bucket of what you might spot when you really look at all the goodness that's happening around you every day. There are more unicorns and rainbows than you might think! It's both exciting and inspiring to know that so many lives are being changed for the positive through these new and unique ways of extending kindness to others. Try taking part or even create your own new idea. You never know the positive impact you may have!

> "KIND WORDS CAN BE SHORT AND EASY TO SPEAK, BUT THEIR ECHOES ARE TRULY ENDLESS."
> –MOTHER TERESA, RENOWNED SAINT AND MISSIONARY

Want a few more ways to spread a little kindness and make a difference? Let Betty show you the way!

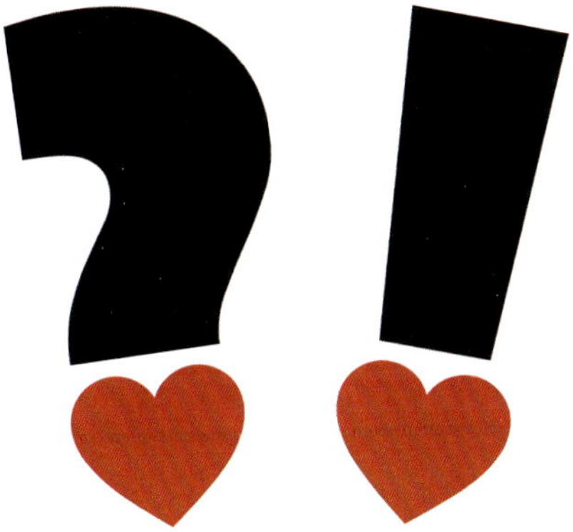

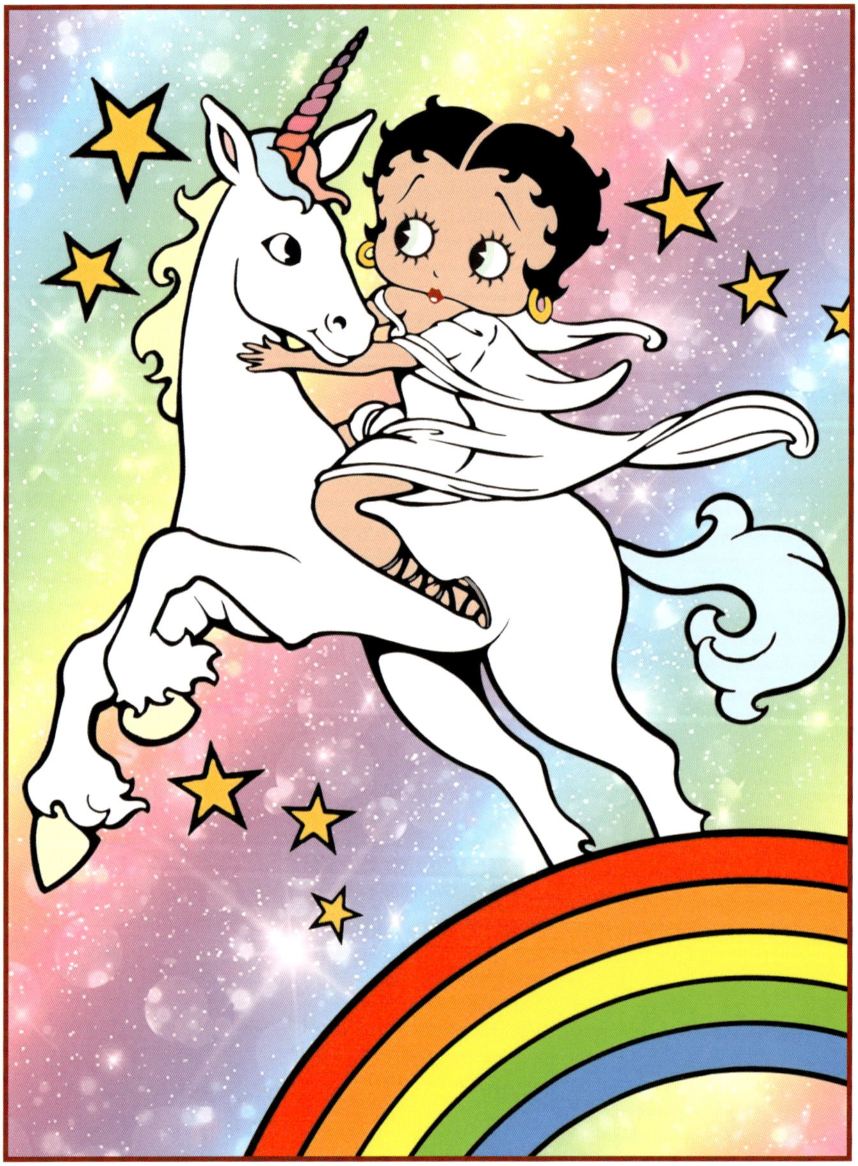

THE PRINCIPLE– Giving of Ourselves Is the Kindest Thing We Can Do

Betty's Inspiration: Volunteering is a victory for everyone!

Become a Reader at Your Local Library or School. There are countless volunteer opportunities at local libraries and schools where you can not only spread kindness and make a difference, you can get a rewarding dose of fun interaction with kids and others in your community who will benefit from the time you're giving. Becoming a reader is a great place to start. Libraries and schools will always welcome your help.

If You're Good at Something, Teach Others. Everyone is great at something, and sharing that knowledge and talent by teaching others is not only a wonderful act of kindness, it's almost an obligation! Wouldn't it be a shame to be the best ukulele player in your county and not share a few tips with someone interested in learning? Maybe your talent is gardening, math, or painting with watercolors. Whatever it is, look for opportunities to share your skills and knowledge. Many local community centers and extension programs look for people to teach a variety of fun courses. You can even start a group or club for people in your community interested in what you have to share. It's all about getting creative!

Spend a Few Hours a Month Serving Meals for a Non-profit. Volunteering to serve meals at a homeless shelter, or to deliver meals for an organization that helps seniors such as Meals on Wheels is a heart-filling experience and fantastic expression of kindness. If you don't have a few hours a month, how about a holiday or two a year? Charitable organizations can always use a helping hand when serving welcome meals on Thanksgiving or Veterans Day. There's something about a hot meal served to someone in need that radiates kindness—from the way it's lovingly prepared to the intention of those who serve it. This is a wonderful thing!

Organize a Canned-Food Drive. This is easy to do and a great way to spread loving kindness in your local community. You can do this simply by partnering with a local food bank or homeless shelter and then spreading the word with friends and neighbors that you're collecting canned foods for that organization. Organize a drop-off day and location and then rally everyone to bring their contributions. You can even work with a local school and get the kids involved in helping out by bringing canned food contributions to school with them on a designated day for collection.

DID YOU KNOW?

The 1938 Betty Boop cartoon *Pudgy and the Lost Kitten* features the work of Lillian Friedman, the first woman to be employed as an animator at Fleischer Studios—or in fact, any traditional animation studio!

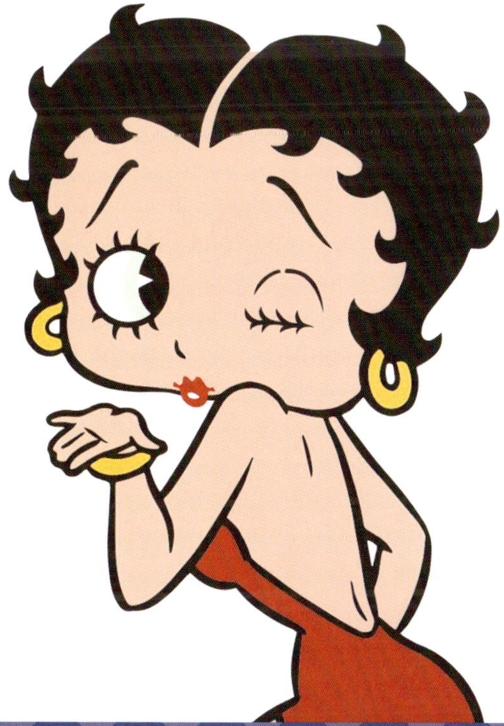

"KINDNESS
IS FREE.
SPREAD IT
WHEREVER
YOU GO."

Chapter 4

Going in Style

Betty Boop has long been known as a style icon. Generations of women have been drawn to her flirty and feminine looks, and celebrities have even channeled her on the red carpet.

In this chapter we'll talk about why Betty's style is so enduring, showcase several of her most iconic fashion moments, and show you multiple ways you can capture the essence of Betty's timeless style and make it your own by incorporating some of her best (and most fun!) tips and tricks into your everyday and special occasion looks.

As one of the original influencers of the 1930s and "It Girls," Betty Boop has provided endless inspiration over the years when it comes to fashion and personal style. Fashion designers have included Betty-inspired looks in countless runway shows, ready-to-wear collections, and high-fashion spectacles. She's been called a style icon, trendsetter, and muse by many in the fashion world.

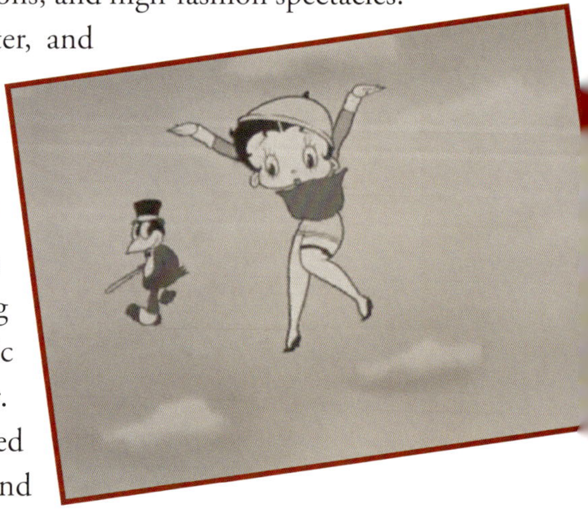

Long before the famous image was cemented in our minds of Marilyn Monroe's dress blowing wildly upward from a subway vent, Betty introduced the iconic pose when her dress was blowing wildly upward from the wind in the classic 1932 cartoon *Betty Boop's Ups and Downs*.

Personal style and fashion have played empowering roles in self-expression and making statements for centuries. A fantastic dress or a great power suit can not only make a statement, it can add to our self-confidence and can-do outlook, making us feel like we can take on the world!

The iconic designer Karl Lagerfeld once said, "Sweatpants are a sign of defeat." Now, while this amusing statement might make you laugh (and, who doesn't love a lazy Sunday in some cozy sweats now and then?), what he's really trying to say through humor is that when you rise to the occasion by dressing for it (and with the right attitude, of course), you can expect the occasion to also rise to you. A great concept to live by—and certainly *very* Betty.

From the flirty flapper styles of the twenties to the flower-filled peace-inspired styles of the sixties to the girl boss power suits of the nineties, Betty has represented them all with panache.

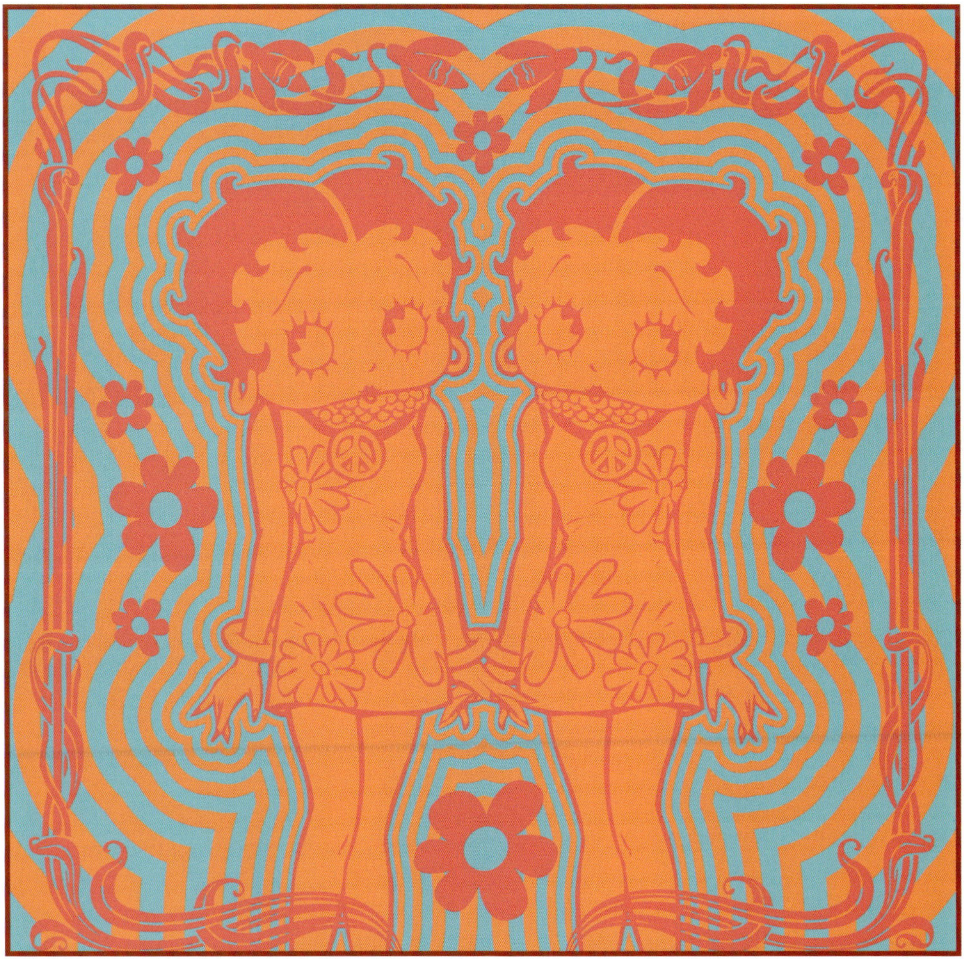

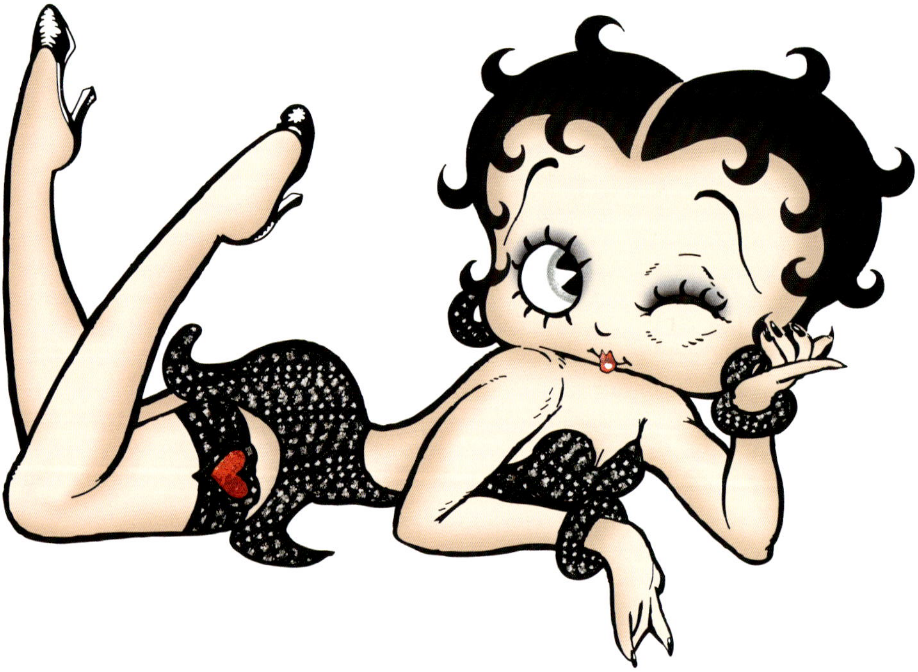

Although she's an animated character, Betty's got such a larger-than-life persona and has had such an impact on pop culture, both past and present, that she is often viewed as a real-life woman. A single girl who loves big city life and dresses for herself (rather than to catch the eye of a guy), she could easily fit right in with the cast of *Friends* and would definitely hang out with the girls from *Sex and the City*.

In 1991, legendary fashion designer Bob Mackie included Betty Boop in a runway fashion show inspired by eight American women he referred to as "remarkable originals of the 20th century with their own particular achievements, style, and charisma." For this show, Betty was in excellent company with her fellow (non-animated!) honorees Diana Vreeland, Billie Holiday, Rita Hayworth, Grace Kelly, Marty Martin, Martha Graham, and Lucille Ball. Each woman was represented by a design inspired by her and worn by one of the day's most popular models. Betty's look included a show-stopping little black beaded flapper-style dress.

In 2013, Betty starred with model Daria Werbowy in a glamorous and fun short film called *Star Eyes* produced by the cosmetic company Lancôme for a mascara campaign. In the popular short, Betty shares tips with her friend Daria about starring on the big screen. In addition to the adorable short, the campaign also featured sparkly images of Betty looking ready for a night on the town with her girlfriends in a dazzling little black dress. Once again, Betty successfully blurred the lines between Cartoon Queen and real life It Girl (a girl we'd all love to hang out with!).

Then, in 2017 prolific fashion designer Zac Posen, known for his feminine silhouettes and sophisticated, glamorous style, created two Betty Boop–inspired dress designs for his collection that captured the essence of her style. Zac is a longtime fan of Betty (and Betty, of course, is a huge fan of Zac's). The collaboration created buzz in the fashion world, received widespread media coverage including a two-page spread in *Marie Claire* magazine, which featured Zac himself and model Crystal Renn posed as Betty showing off the chic red dresses.

As part of the celebration of the new designs, Zac and Betty also starred in their own all-new animated short film called *Betty Goes A-Posen*—which of course made a big splash on YouTube.

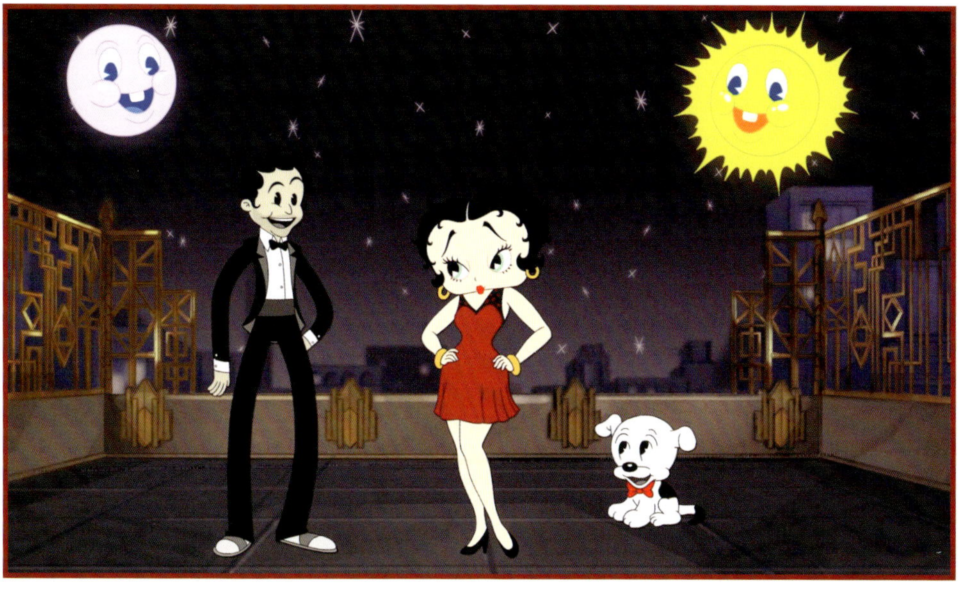

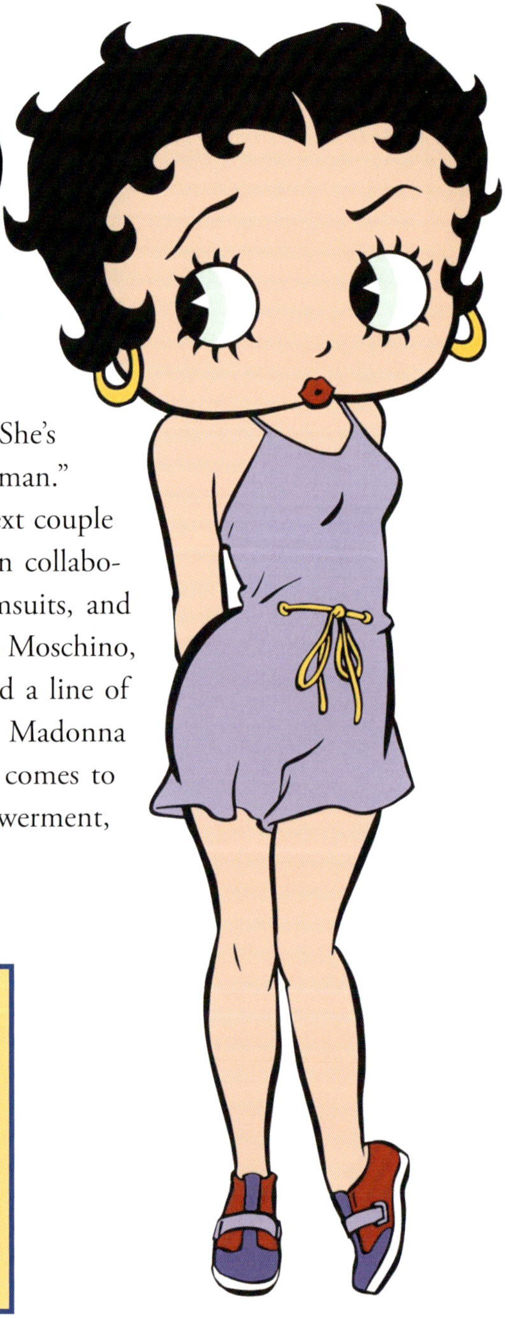

"In many ways, I think Betty is more poignant than ever, because she's in sync with this idea of a femme fatale feminist—the idea that you can possess feminine attributes but not be defined by your sexuality," Posen told *Marie Claire*. "She's not a blow-up doll; she's an independent woman."

Following the Zac Posen designs, the next couple of years were filled with high-profile fashion collaborations for Betty, including handbags, swimsuits, and apparel featuring Betty's iconic likeness from Moschino, designs from streetwear brand Supreme, and a line of tee shirts with a cult following (including Madonna herself!) from Yves Saint Laurent. When it comes to fashion, femininity, and personal empowerment, Betty continues to inspire.

"THE BEST COLOR IN THE WHOLE WORLD IS THE ONE THAT LOOKS GOOD ON YOU."

–COCO CHANEL, LEGENDARY DESIGNER

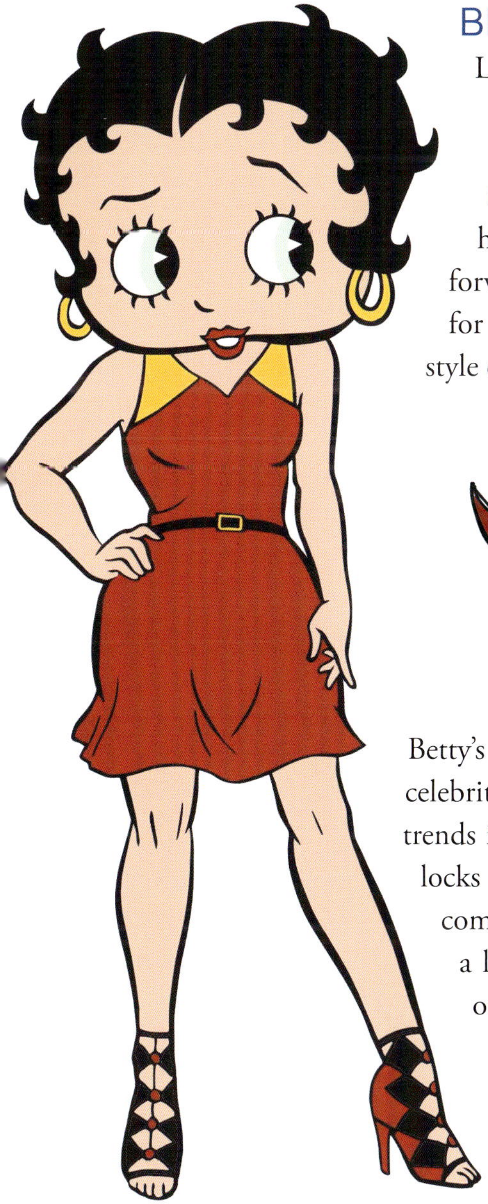

BETTY'S SIGNATURE LOOK

Like any well-informed fashion girl, Betty knows that the secret to great style is a simplified closet full of go-to signature pieces with a few trends mixed in for good measure. Betty has been seen over the years in many fashion-forward looks, but she's become most recognized for her fun, timeless signature style. A few of the style elements she's most known for include:

- Little black or red dress
- Gold hoop earrings
- Red or black heels
- Long, feminine lashes
- Sweet brunette curls

Betty's signature look has been channeled by countless celebrities on the red carpet, and continues to influence trends in both fashion and beauty. Betty's short, curly locks are constantly being referenced online when comparing celebrity hairstyles, and you'll rarely see a little red dress on the runway without a media outlet (or ten!) comparing it to Betty Boop.

In May 2019, Betty Boop was celebrated by *Vogue* magazine as one of 25 "Camp Beauty Icons," along with stars such as Josephine Baker, Cher, Grace Jones, Mae West, Marilyn Monroe, Rihanna, and more in a story highlighting the theme of the 2019 Met Gala, *Camp: Notes on Fashion*. The magazine noted that Cupid's bow-lipped Betty "bucked tradition and set the stage for pure liberated beauty."

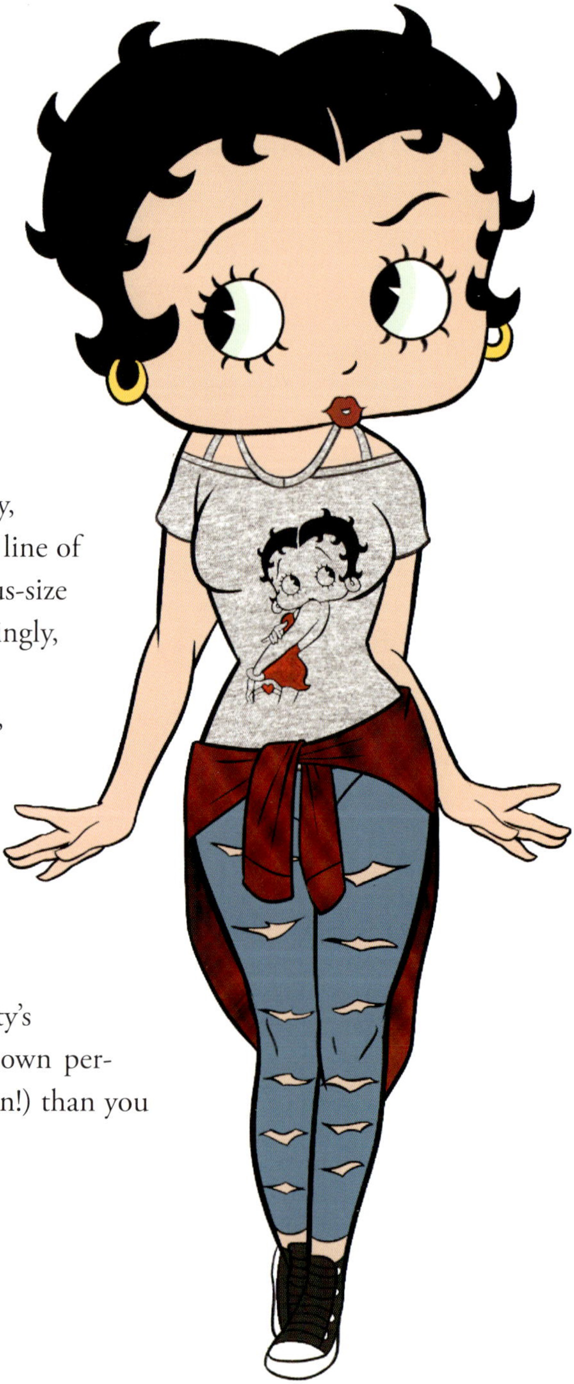

Betty also is regularly praised for not being afraid to show off her curves with her form-fitting choices. This was celebrated when she was chosen in 2018 to be the muse for an entire episode of the hit Bravo fashion design series, *Project Runway All Stars*, where some of the show's top all-star designers created looks inspired by Betty, with the winner, Joshua McKinley, receiving the honor of designing a line of Betty Boop pieces for leading plus-size fashion retailer Torrid. Not surprisingly, the designs quickly sold out.

Despite Betty's fabulousness, she is not high-maintenance. She actually manages to keep up her glamorous persona with a few simple principles that can be easily followed by anyone who might be inspired. So, how can you incorporate Betty's signature low-fuss vibe into your own personal style? It's easier (and more fun!) than you may think!

THE PRINCIPLE– Betty's Rules of Style

Betty's Inspiration: Fashion and personal style can be both fun and empowering.

Keep Things Simple. You'll never see Betty wearing more than just a few easy pieces. She doesn't have too many things in her closet. Just a few favorites she can mix and match, with the occasional trend mixed in. At times, you'll see her in just a little dress and heels. She wears very little jewelry, but what she does wear makes a statement. She'll be the first to tell you that the secret to making any outfit more fabulous is hoop earrings!

Limit the Trends. Choosing just one key trend per season that will seamlessly fit in with your classics is not only a good style strategy, it's budget-friendly too. Simplifying your closet with a few good quality classics is a very Betty approach (and will make your life easier).

Have a Signature Dress. You'll often see Betty in a little black or red dress. A simple little dress can become your wardrobe BFF! The perfect dress for you will be one you feel comfortable in, flatters your body type, and fits you absolutely perfectly (don't be afraid to have it professionally tailored—it's worth it). It will be a dress that can take you from day to night and brunch to dinner. Just change up the shoes and jewelry to create different looks. Add a favorite jacket or coat, a hat or scarf, and just like Betty you'll be ready for whatever weather comes your way.

Focus on Classics. Like Betty's signature dress, the rest of her closet is made up of easy classics she can put together in a flash. A good fitting pair of jeans, a pencil skirt or two, a couple easy blouses, a few cute but comfy loungewear pieces such as leggings and sweatshirts (perfect for yoga or a lazy Sunday), sneakers, sandals, and a couple pairs of fierce and fabulous heels. A wardrobe focused on classics is both timeless and easy on the purse strings.

Choose Handbags Wisely. When it comes to handbags, rather than spend her entire budget on a whole bunch of different bags, Betty would rather use that budget to buy just one high quality bag that will last for years. With this strategy (possibly buying just one new handbag every year or two), one can build a great capsule collection of very nice bags (that never go out of style!) over time. If you've wondered how that stylish friend of yours affords those high-quality bags she carries, this could be the secret. This same concept applies when it comes to wardrobe classics overall. Investing in quality over quantity is the key to a beautifully curated minimalist closet full of fabulous finds and signature style pieces! So Betty!

Have a Go-To Hairstyle. A signature hairstyle that works great for you will make getting ready a breeze. Betty's flirty, fun curly locks flatter her face and are always in style. A great stylist can look at your hair color, texture, and the shape of your face and recommend a cut that will look amazing on you. Try going to your stylist and without giving any direction, simply ask what they recommend. Believe us when we tell you this can be life changing!

Identify the Hair Products Designed for You. Once you find that great cut that works perfectly for you, invest in the products to keep it up and see if you can learn to style it in under ten minutes (more time for special occasions, of course). A good hair day will help fuel confidence and make you feel fab, and with a go-to style that's easy to maintain, you can have many more of them!

PUSHING STYLE BOUNDARIES

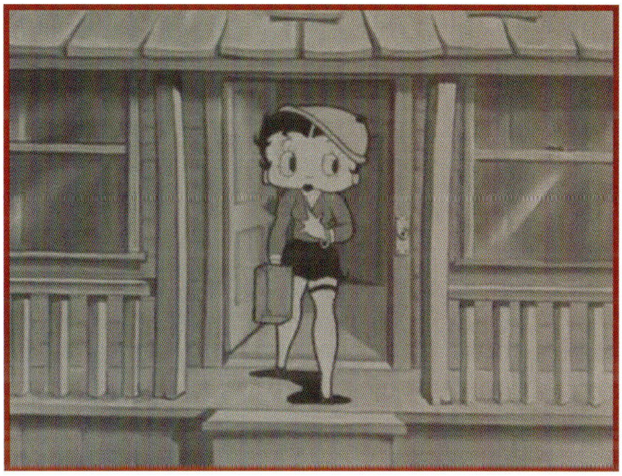

There's one principle of style that Betty has always embraced that we definitely need to elaborate on here, and that's pushing boundaries. Betty has never been afraid to do this, but at times it's been a challenge for her to stay true to herself (can you relate?).

Remember that little thing called The Motion Picture Production Code we mentioned earlier? Also known as the Hays Code, it was established to determine and regulate what content and imagery was considered "acceptable" for public audiences in motion pictures produced in the United States. This greatly affected Betty Boop, as the conservative administrators appointed to enforce the code were not fans of Betty's short dresses and flirty style. As a result, by the mid-thirties, the animators at Fleischer Studios were forced to "tone down" Betty's appearance (and even bits of her personality!), putting her in more modest outfits that included longer skirts and other more conservative looks.

In spite of these attempts to "quiet" Betty's voice, she rose to even further fame, becoming one of the most famous and beloved animated characters on the big screen. Her style was still fabulous, and she was still taking on important issues in her own unique ways.

Over that next twenty years, the Hays Code was followed, but grew to be fairly unpopular, and by the late 1950s, producers and directors began to ignore the regulations and the popularity of television added to the challenges of enforcing the code. After many years of little to no enforcement, the code was nixed in 1968 and replaced with the modern-day film rating system.

VIEW STYLE AS A WAY OF LIFE

In the 1934 cartoon *Keep in Style*, Betty hosts her own expo where she showcases the latest innovations from cars to kitchen appliances that are designed to make life easier and more fun. She implies that style is all in the attitude.

In the same cartoon, Betty also sings about how being creative with what you've already got can "help you keep in style." Sounds budget-friendly too, right? She sings and dances before the cheering audience while she reinvents the outfit she's wearing right before their eyes. She removes the sleeves from her blouse and transforms them into ruffles around her ankles, then struts across the stage showing them off. Soon, the look becomes a new trend across the nation with all the fashionable women (and men!) showing off the look. Instagram-worthy for sure!

It will cost you but a trifle
You can give your friends an eyeful
If you want to keep in style
Take the things you have and change them
You just have to re-arrange them
And you'll always keep in style . . . You don't have to be a big millionaire
You can show them that you know what to wear
Put a little zip and dashin'
To your smile for it's the fashion
And you'll always be in style!

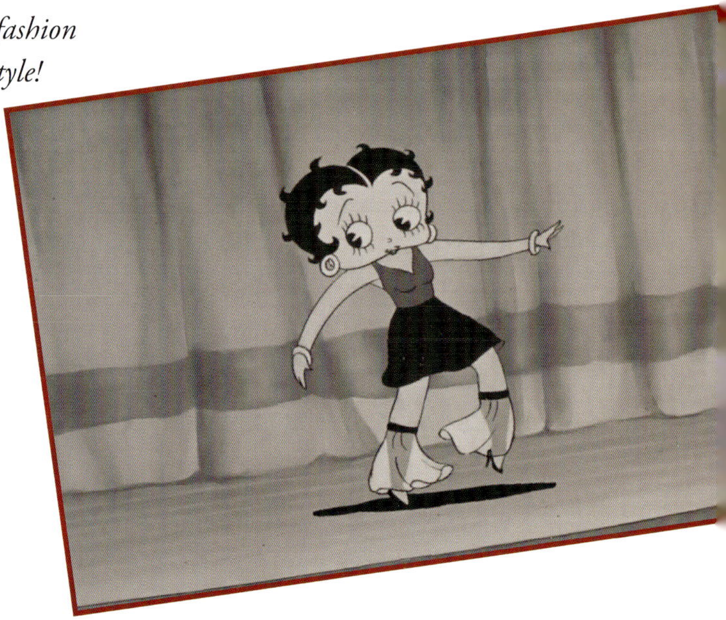

> "STYLE IS SOMETHING EACH OF US ALREADY HAS, ALL WE NEED TO DO IS FIND IT."
> –DIANE VON FURSTENBERG, FASHION DESIGNER AND WOMEN'S EMPOWERMENT ADVOCATE

In many ways, style is all about how *you* look at it and incorporate it into your everyday life. It's a fun way to showcase who you are and tell the world a little about yourself without having to say a word.

THE PRINCIPLE–Tricks of the Trade

Betty's Inspiration: We not only want to look good, we want to feel good.

If the Shoe Fits . . . Clearing your closet of any shoes that hurt your feet is a must. Nobody can feel their best with squished toes or blisters. Maybe you bought a pair a half-size too small because they were on sale? It's time to say goodbye and donate them to a fashionista they'll fit.

Show Your Legs and Feet a Little Support. This is especially important if you're pounding the pavement all day or settling in for a long flight. If your feet or ankles get sore, tired, or swollen after a long day, try compression socks or comfy socks with some arch support. They actually make some that are very stylish and they're worth every penny!

Let Your Clothes Breathe. Cottons, linens, cashmere, and other natural fabrics need to breathe to keep their shape and stay fresh. Stuffing them in the back of the closet for months on end can result in yellowing, moth holes, hard-to-remove wrinkles, and more yucky stuff. Taking them out every few weeks, reshaping them, hanging them in the fresh air for a bit, and addressing stains and spots will give these garments a longer life—and will make sure you always look your best.

Layers Will Take You from Morning to Evening. Layering is every fashion girl's secret for going from day to evening, especially between seasons when it can be chilly in the morning and hot in the afternoon. A light cardigan or blazer over your go-to dress can be removed in the evening to take you from the office to cocktails with ease. A dressy top under a pantsuit will take you from that office meeting to that office party. And, by removing the blazer and adding a statement necklace, you're ready for an evening out. Plus, layering is fun! Who doesn't like two outfits in one? Your friends will marvel at how well put together you are (and you'll smile at how easy it is!).

Stay Cozy When on the Go. Always be sure to travel with a shawl or a wrap in your carry-on bag when you travel; you'll thank yourself when the plane or hotel is chilly. It's also a good idea to pack a pair of comfortable flats you can change into if your feet start to ache or you find yourself walking an unexpected distance.

Don't Underrate the Underwear. Do you know what the number one secret is on Hollywood red carpets? It's not the gowns or accessories . . . it's the undergarments! Any stylist to the stars will tell you that shape garments are key to looking fabulous in your favorite outfits. Good-fitting shape wear can help pull you in where you need it, offer support for your back, and accentuate curves in all the right places.

Let's Hear It for "The Girls." Good bras and camisoles can improve posture and add definition under a blouse or sweater. The proper fit can literally transform your figure! Plus, when you're supported in all the right places, you can't help but glow from within from the added confidence and assurance you feel. Many lingerie stores offer free bra fittings with a professional to help you find just the right fit for you. The right underthings can make a tremendous difference when it comes to looking and feeling fabulous!

STYLE THROUGH THE AGES

Fashion, makeup, and ever-changing trends are nothing new. Even the ancient Egyptians had style! In fact, they even wore some of the fabrics and cuts that we still wear today, including linen, maxi-dresses, and pleats. They wore show-stopping jewelry they believed showed off their wealth and to appear more showy and attractive to the Gods. But it wasn't just the wealthy women who wore jewelry. Fun, affordable jewelry was sometimes made from colorful pottery beads.

Women in ancient Egypt even wore makeup. They got creative with natural elements such as minerals and plants, using kohl as eyeliner and colored powders on the eyelids and cheeks. Kohl around the eyes provided some sun protection and also was believed to protect one from evil. Many women wore makeup daily and felt empowered by it!

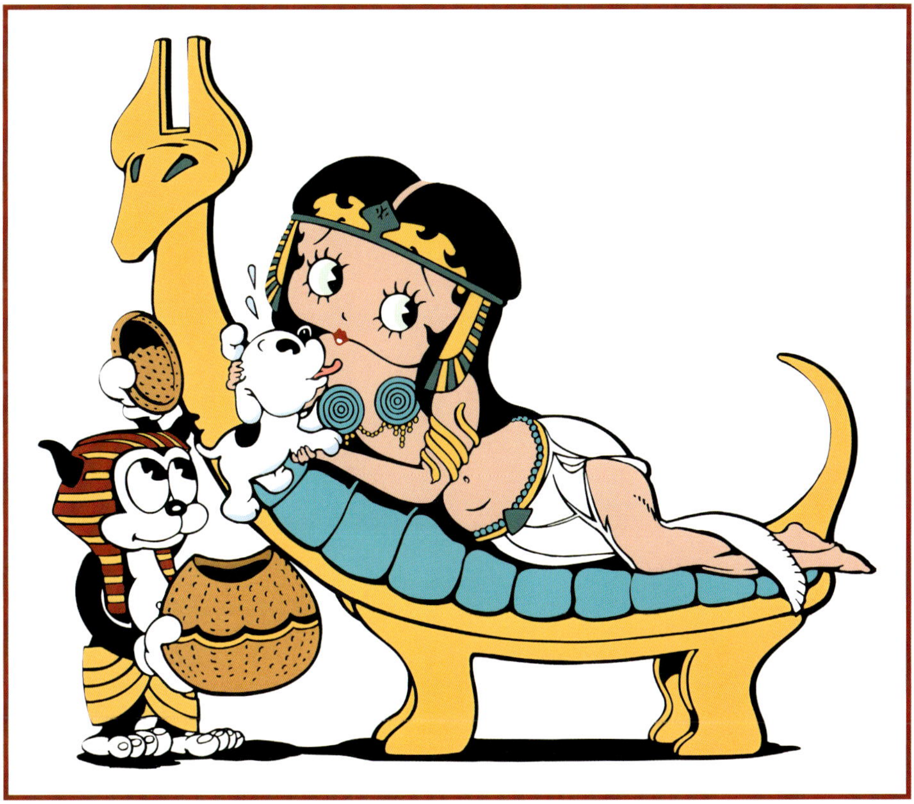

In another ancient society, ancient Greeks wore body-conscious, draped clothing that was super comfortable and provided sun protection. Some wore bright colored fabrics to show status, as it wasn't cheap to dye clothing back then. They carried small purses on their belts (the original belt-bag!) that smartly, were sometimes hidden.

In fact, when it comes to purses, they've actually been used by both men and women throughout the course of history for thousands of years! While today they hold everything from lipstick to keys to a passport, in ancient times they held everything from food to tools to weapons.

As time went on, fashion became less practical and even more about self-expression and status. Gowns, jewels, boots, sandals, makeup, handbags—they've all had their place throughout fashion history and still continue to evolve through time, while remaining largely the same.

Did you know that high-heeled shoes were originally worn by men? They were created as early as the tenth century to help warriors stay on horses, but after time became fashionable for men, especially kings and courtiers. It wasn't until hundreds of years later that the first instance of a woman wearing high heels was noted when Italian noblewoman Catherine de Medici wore a pair at her wedding to King Henry II of France so she could appear taller!

Even after de Medici wore heels for her wedding, their allure faded with women while remaining somewhat popular with men. Yet, two centuries later they really took off again as a status symbol among royals and noblemen in the French court during the time of Louis XIV (who wore his own special red pair). It wasn't until much later, however, that heels became really popular with women. In fact, the famous stiletto heel wasn't even invented until the early nineteenth century. Many women today (including Betty!) are sure happy they were!

While fashion changes and trends come and go, one thing remains the same—classics are classics! And, Betty Boop definitely knows how to embrace them. What better way to have fun with classics than by adding a little *Boop* to your closet?

YOUR BETTY BOOP–INSPIRED CAPSULE WARDROBE

As a fun resource and a little added inspiration, we've created a guide to help you put together your very own Betty Boop–inspired capsule wardrobe. You can customize as needed of course, but this is a creative way to bring a bit of Betty into your own signature style.

The List:

Little Red Dress
Little Black Dress
A Classic Polka-Dot Dress
Gold Hoop Earrings
Classic Black Pumps
Classic Red Pumps
Little Beaded Handbag (Red or Black)
Timeless Carry-All Handbag
Black-and-White Polka-Dot Blouse
Faux Fur Jacket (Betty never wears real fur)
Red Nail and Lip

FASHION AND SELF-EXPRESSION

Earlier, we touched on how fashion and personal style can play an important role in self-expression for women. From stand-out bright colors to power suits to funky hairs-dos, your style can be the first thing that shows the world who you are and what you're all about!

Betty Boop's personal style is associated with fun, confidence, femininity, and sass. What a compliment it is to be known as the Original Sass Symbol! Her style is so recognized that it's regularly cited in fashion pages when describing celebrities on the red carpet that are donning short curly locks, flirty dresses, and red pouty lips. Betty's signature look has become a *go-to* for women who want to project the vibes that the look stands for.

When you think of women with standout signature style, who (besides Betty, of course) comes to mind? We can think of several right away: Phyllis Diller, Jackie O, Iris Apfel, Madonna, and Lady Gaga, just to name a few.

How would you describe your sense of style? Does it reflect who you are and support the way you want to feel? Are there small changes you might make that would add some additional fun and inspiration? Try creating some fresh looks with what's already in your closet. Mix, match, twirl in front of the mirror, and most of all have fun with it!

THE PRINCIPLE– Looking Your Best Every Day

Betty's Inspiration: Simple little tricks will help you look your best, even on the busiest days.

Forget the Clumpy Mascara. If your mascara isn't working for you, don't hesitate to throw it out. Spider lashes or clumps don't flatter anyone. There are so many high-quality choices. In fact, many makeup artists will tell you they don't have to be expensive! Some of their favorites can be purchased right in your local drug store.

Choose Makeup That's Right for Your Complexion. When it comes to foundation or concealer, a good rule to follow is to match it to your neck, not your face. This works very well for seamless color. We've all seen ladies with unfortunate orange spots on their faces from mis-matched concealer. Don't be one of them. And, when applying foundation and blush, apply in down strokes so all that little peach fuzz doesn't stick straight up.

Try This Fabulous Lip Tip. For full, pouty lips like Betty's, try lining and filling in your entire lip with a pencil that matches your natural lip color. Then apply lipstick or gloss. This even foundation will give the appearance of fabulous, full lips and avoid the "leftover line" look after the lipstick wears off.

Choose the Right Earrings. Did you know that shiny earrings that reflect light also will light up your eyes? You don't need many pairs. In fact, just one favorite pair will do! Betty is almost always seen wearing her favorite gold hoop earrings that are both flattering and classic.

A Bright Smile Says It All. Keeping your pearly whites shiny and bright has never been easier! There are some wonderful and affordable teeth-whitening products available right in your local drugstore and they take only a few minutes a week. Your smile is your very best accessory, and if you care for it, it will last you a lifetime (unlike most things in your closet!). Find a product that's right for you (ask your dentist if you're not sure) and give it a try. You'll be amazed at the difference just a few treatments can make!

STYLE ON A BUDGET

It's important to remember that style is an attitude, an expression. It's about what works for you and makes you feel like the fabulous woman you are. It's not about how much you spend! Some of the most glamorous women in the world stick with classics they've had in their closets for years. French women, known for their impeccable sense of chic, are known for shopping at thrift stores and flea markets for one-of-a-kind finds and classics alike!

In fact, by shopping at secondhand boutiques, online auction sites, and thrift stores, you can sometimes find high quality fabrics, shoes, and even designer labels for a tiny fraction of what they would cost in a department store. Plus, it's fun! Who doesn't love a fashion treasure hunt? Not to mention, buying clothing secondhand is good for the environment. Reduce, reuse, and recycle—even when it comes to fashion!

Another fun idea for budget-friendly style is to host a clothing exchange party with all your friends. Have everyone go through their closets for things that no longer fit or work for them and bring the clean items that are in good shape to your place for a fun night of trading and cocktails! What a great idea for freshening up your wardrobe while having fun with the girls!

Finally, remember that fashion and personal style isn't about showcasing a particular item (although this can be fun!), it's about showcasing *you!* You are a fun, fierce, and fabulous female and a force to be recognized! Always remember this and be true to yourself. And before you know it, you won't be following the trends, you'll be setting the trends!

DID YOU KNOW?

Betty Boop's persona was inspired by many jazz-age influencers—flappers and singers of the 1920s—but contrary to popular belief, was not directly inspired by any one single performer.

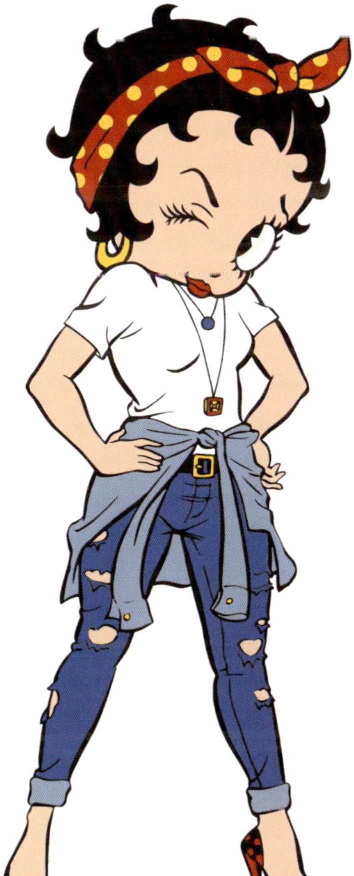

"ATTITUDE IS EVERYTHING!"

Chapter 5

Accentuate the Positive

One of the things fans love most about Betty is that she always finds positive solutions and maintains an overall positive outlook in almost any situation. She's an optimist without being unrealistic. She'll point out what's good or what *can* be done (instead of what can't) and then take action to do it. She's always focused on solutions.

Not everyone is naturally positive or optimistic, but everyone can train himself or herself to be more naturally positive with practice. It just takes focusing with intent on being positive for a long enough period (roughly a month for most people) and you'll literally re-train your "mind muscles" to stay on the sunny side more naturally. And, it's definitely worth the effort. Not only will you be happier overall, you'll likely live even longer and healthier!

POSITIVITY AND YOUR WELL-BEING

We all know that when we're keeping a positive outlook, we feel better overall—physically and mentally—about a situation. There are many good reasons for this. According to numerous high-profile studies, optimism and positivity are actually vitally important to overall health. Research has shown that optimism can reduce risk of hypertension, infections, stress, fatigue, depression, and heart disease.

In one study, researchers from Harvard and Boston University evaluated 1,306 male volunteers with an average age of sixty-one. Each volunteer was reviewed to see whether their outlook and explanatory style was optimistic or pessimistic, and then their overall health was evaluated, including obesity, blood pressure, alcohol use, smoking habits, and family history of heart disease. None of the volunteers had been diagnosed with coronary artery disease at the beginning of the ten-year study. At the end of the ten years, the study found that the most pessimistic men were more than twice as likely to develop heart disease than those with the optimistic, positive outlook, even after they took the other risk factors into account. Over twice as likely! Aren't those results amazing?

Here's a fun and interesting bit of information on positivity to share with the sports fans in your life. A 1988 French study on cardiovascular mortality found that it's possible the boost of optimism sports fans experience when their team wins may result in fewer heart attacks.

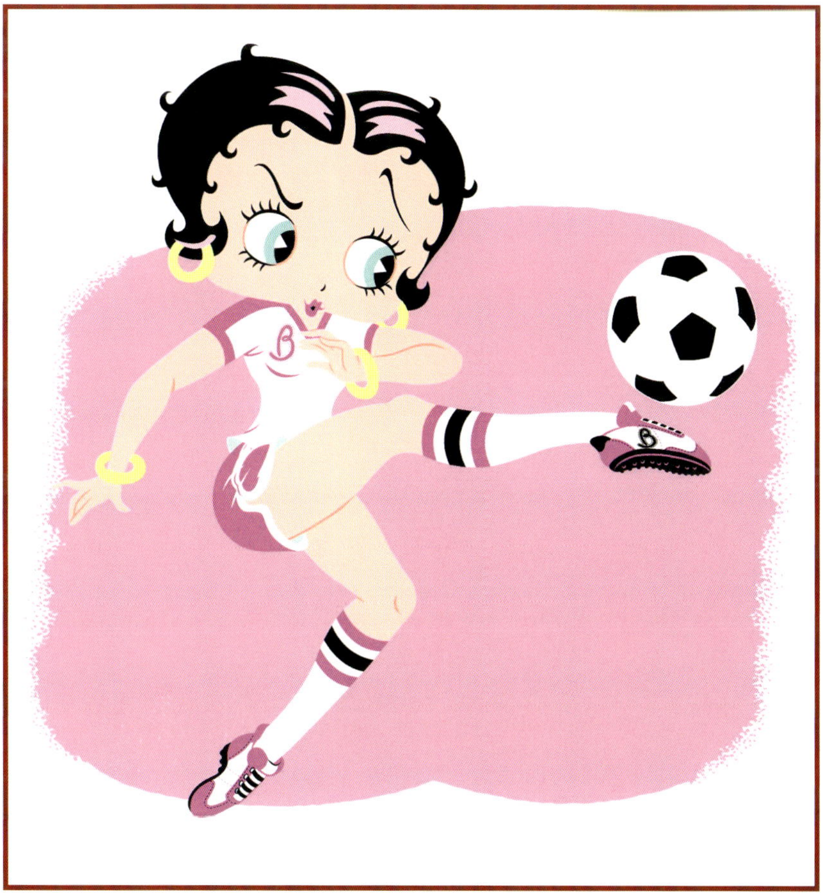

On July 12th of that year, France beat Brazil in the World Cup of soccer, which at the time was the biggest sporting event ever held in France. In looking at records of cardiovascular deaths between the dates of July 7th and 17th of that year, researchers found that French men suffered fewer fatal heart attacks on Game Day than on any of the other days, whereas French women did not. Perhaps this suggests that all the good feelings the guys enjoyed while cheering for their team also were great for the health of their hearts. Good thing Betty is a sports fan!

TRAIN YOURSELF TO LIVE A MORE POSITIVE LIFE

Yes, even if you tend to be on the pessimistic side, you can actually create new habits and train yourself to be more naturally positive! Think of it as a sort of "diet" for the mind. Positive thinking will not only make you happier and healthier overall, it will help you attract more positive relationships into your life (we'll talk more about that shortly).

The idea here is not to be positive 24/7 (that would make you a robot instead of a human!). It's unrealistic to expect anyone to be upbeat and positive all the time. But, it is realistic to greatly increase one's overall positive thinking and energy. A fantastic goal for sure!

There are numerous ways to train yourself to be more optimistic and have more positive energy in your life. Let's talk about a few proven strategies that will help you get started.

> "KEEP YOUR FACE TO THE SUNSHINE AND YOU CANNOT SEE A SHADOW."
> –HELEN KELLER, AUTHOR

THE PRINCIPLE– Creating More Positivity

Betty's Inspiration: Focusing on the positive will take you far in life.

Learn to Catch Yourself in the Negative. Part of becoming a more positive person is in learning to catch yourself when you're being unnecessarily negative. We can all fall into the space of being a naysayer or doubter now and then, but we also can learn to catch ourselves and make a shift back to the positive when needed. This will not only lift your spirits to a better place, but will boost the positivity of those around you as well.

Believe It and You'll Achieve It. Half of what's involved in accomplishing anything is *believing you can.* Starting off any goal or project with a positive, will-do outlook can make all the difference! When Betty sets out to take care of business, it's because she really believes in herself and what she's doing. You can see it in the way she walks. You can see it on her face. Self-doubt is nowhere to be found. And, you can do the same!

Keep Your Sunny Side Up. This one may be a bit obvious, but it's worth pointing out; training yourself to always look for silver linings about situations can actually seem to help create more of them because they'll be that much more prominent to you. Positivity is a habit, and not everyone possesses it naturally, but we can all adopt it as a skill much in the same way we'd learn to speak a new language. With practice and dedication (just like creating any new habit), anyone can become an optimist and benefit from all the goodness that comes with it.

SURROUND YOURSELF WITH POSITIVE PEOPLE

In Betty's 1936 cartoon, *Making Friends*, she sings an adorable song to Pudgy when he's feeling a bit down:

You gotta have some recreation,
so put yourself in circulation,
go out and make friends with the
world!

If you will only learn to mingle,
your little heart with joy will tingle,
go out and make friends with the
world!

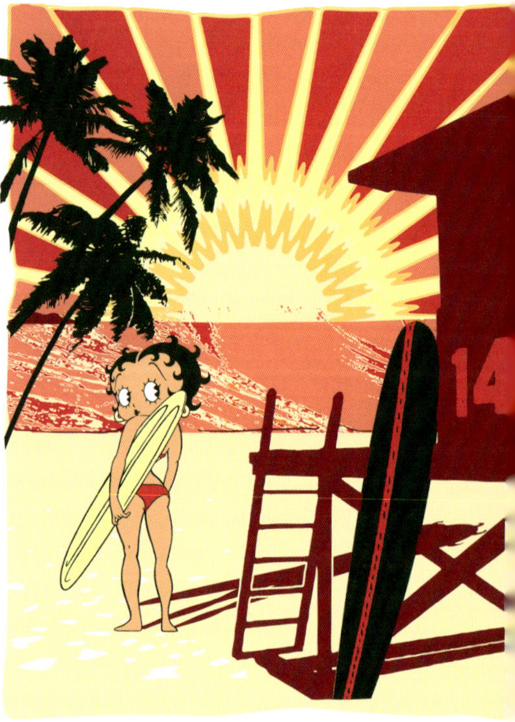

Pudgy takes Betty's advice and ventures out to make some new friends. The joy and positivity shared between Pudgy and his new animal friends as they play together and help each other with tasks is both sweet and mood changing.

Betty's great advice to Pudgy has even been demonstrated by science. A 2010 review by Utah's Brigham Young University of 148 previous studies on social links and mortality found that healthy social ties have as much of a positive impact on lifespan as exercise, and is equal to quitting smoking. That's powerful stuff!

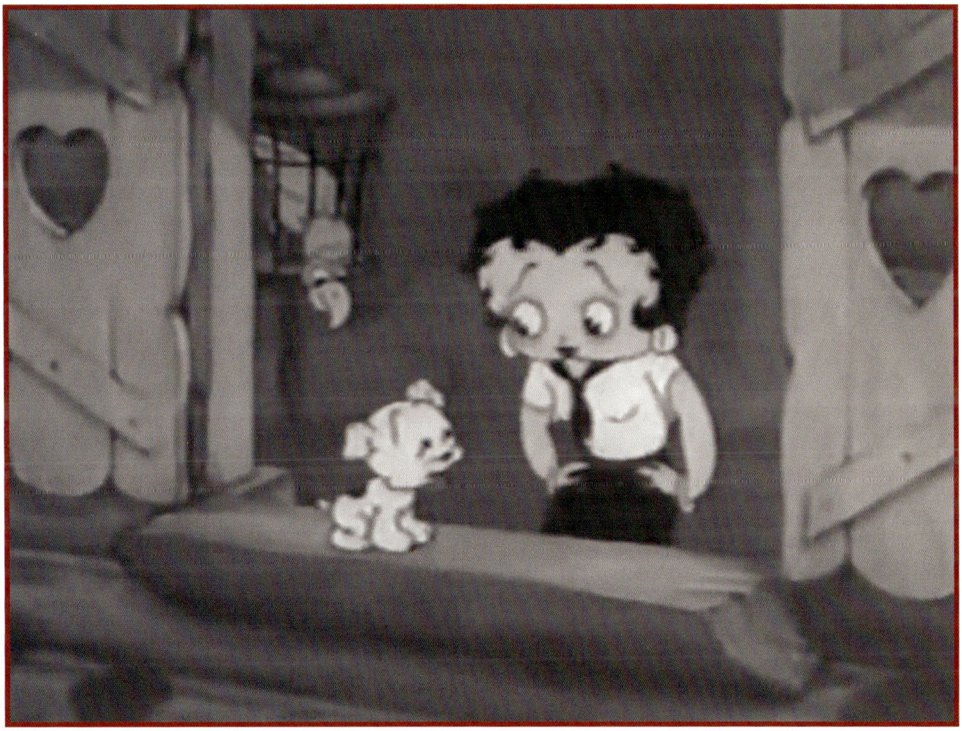

As Pudgy learned, one sure way to surround yourself with positive, uplifting people is to get out and meet more of them. Taking part in groups or community events where they're likely to be is a great way to have some fun and meet your goal of making a few optimistic new friends! You may find groups of like-minded positive people through your church, local chamber of commerce, community center, or even on websites like Meetup. If there's an activity or craft you enjoy, looking for groups centered on those things is a great way to start. You also can sign up as a volunteer for a charity you believe in (Betty loves helping animals).

Another great way to approach cultivating great relationships it is to purposefully schedule more one-on-one time with positive people who inspire you. Create a list of people you know that you'd like to spend more time with or get to know even better (because they're awesome!). Then, take out your calendar and try to schedule a lunch or dinner with at least one per month (two is even better!). Or, create a standing lunch or brunch date with a small handful of these friends. You'll find yourself looking forward to the quality time and to the burst of positive inspiration you'll feel as a result!

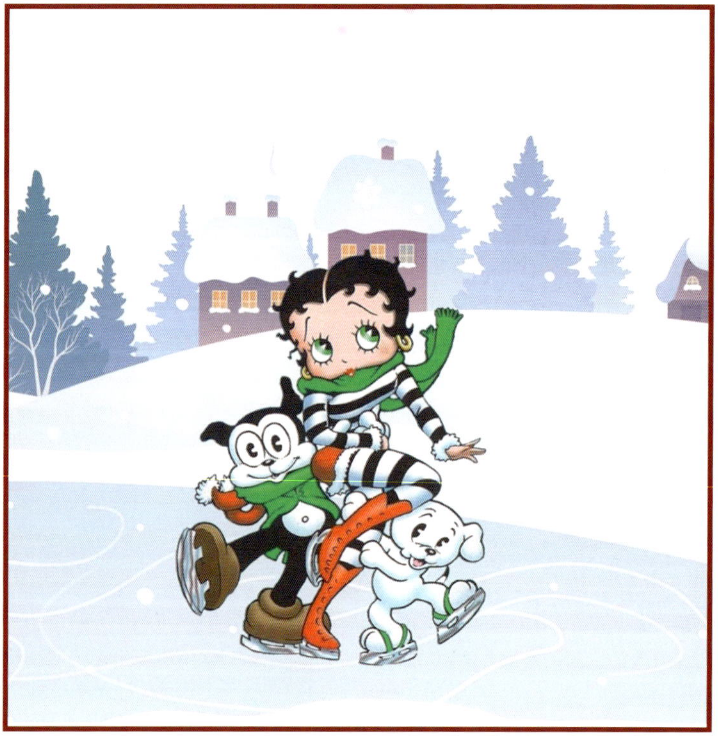

CHANGE UP YOUR MORNINGS

The way you start your day is the way you will live your day. If you start your day off in positive ways (eat right, hydrate, reduce or eliminate stress, don't rush, move your body, and incorporate some kind of positive reading or listening), you'll find that you create solid foundations for more joyful, positive days!

We all know what kind of day we can have if we start off on the wrong side of the bed. Grouchy thoughts, junk food, negative news, too much caffeine, and a variety of other things we know aren't great for us. The negative energy and consequences from that stuff stays with us throughout the day and affect everything we experience. A simple evaluation of how we regularly spend our mornings and then making simple changes to make them more supportive and positive can make a huge difference!

Here's a simple exercise to begin your morning makeover. Create a list of five things you're aware of that you know are unhealthy or draining your positive energy in the mornings. Be very honest with yourself. These can be foods you're eating, bad habits you'd like to ditch, not getting enough sleep, not giving yourself enough time, etc. Once you have this list, create another list with five positive items you can replace those things with that you know will be helpful. They can be very simple and doable, such as cutting back from three cups of coffee to one, going to bed thirty minutes earlier, or replacing a sugary pastry with a piece of fruit. Once you have your lists, they become great visual tools to help you achieve those goals. Then, close your eyes and imagine Betty coaching you through these small changes (you'll smile immediately!), and set your mind to making them happen.

BE DELIBERATELY POSITIVE

Yes, being very deliberate about approaching things (especially challenging things!) in a positive way is a valuable life strategy! It can be easy to be a naysayer or think of all the bad things that might happen if you take that leap, try that new thing, or take on a big project. But it's important to remember that positive thinking is the most important brick in the foundation for anything you do.

Science has shown that positive thinking can literally make your brain function better, and purposeful practices such as positive visualization around different situations can lead to more happiness and success. In a 2016 positive thinking study, researchers from King's College in London tested 102 people who suffered from generalized anxiety disorder. They asked one group to think of three worries that they'd had in the past week and deliberately visualize an *image* of a positive outcome, another part of the group to think of *verbal* positive outcomes, and the last of the group to simply visualize any positive *image* whenever they started to worry. The two groups that used *imagery* in their visualizations reported more decreased anxiety, more happiness, and more restfulness than the group that only pictured verbal outcomes.

It's not that visualizing the verbal outcome didn't help too (all positivity offers a boost), but this study definitely showed the power of picturing actual imagery when it comes to your positive thinking. Try practicing this regularly and you'll create a fantastic new habit!

THE PRINCIPLE– Simple Positivity Tips

Betty's Inspiration: Adding positivity to daily life is as simple as A, B, C.

Do a TV Cleanse. Go through what's on your watch lists and what shows you're saving or recording. Delete any that don't make you feel uplifted in some way. Believe it or not, watching violent, negative shows can lead to more negativity in other areas of your life (especially in your dreams!). Once you've deleted any negative shows you no longer need in your life, go through and see what you might find in the genres of comedy, romance, and family entertainment. Find a few that make you smile or spark your interest and add them to your watch list or set them to record. Now, you'll always have something uplifting to watch that creates positive vibes!

Surround Yourself with Positivity Boosters. Believe it or not, small things can make a big difference. Fresh flowers, strategically placed sticky notes with positive phrases, and having your favorite healthy breakfast options on hand to start your day are all ideas for sprinkling your life with things that can help boost your mood and positivity. Try creating a list of little things you can do to boost your positivity factor.

Set a Daily Reminder on Your Smartphone. Did you know you can use the alarm setting on your smartphone for more than just wake-up calls? Most phones will allow you to label alarms with little reminder notes with each alarm you set. So, your morning alarm may be labeled with a note to yourself that says, "Good morning! Coffee time! Make it a great day!" Then, each morning you'll see this little reminder. A nice way to start the day! You also might try setting a daily alarm in the afternoon labeled with a reminder to stretch and get some fresh air.

REDUCING NEGATIVITY IN YOUR LIFE

You may have noticed it's possible to "catch" positivity or negativity much like catching a cold. If you're around bright, positive people you'll feel more positive yourself (plus, you'll feel great!). On the flip side, we all know what it's like to hang out with negative, pessimistic people (perhaps some are family members), and how it can put you in a bad mood and seem to drain the life out of you.

The same concept goes for media and entertainment on which we choose to focus. There is so much violence and negativity in entertainment and in the news today, it can really bring you down if you don't carefully guard what's invading your space! A practice of simply becoming more deliberate about choosing positive and uplifting content to enjoy when watching TV, movies, or reading books can make a big difference. At the same time, turning the channel or skipping over anything you know will bring you down is excellent self-care and a very powerful practice for reducing negativity in your life to make room for much better stuff!

Another factor that we may not even realize could be adding negativity to our lives involves the places in which we spend our time. Are the rooms or buildings you spend time in cluttered, dark, or draining in some way? Are you finding yourself regularly in spaces that bring you down, rather than inspire? It's very easy to underestimate how significantly the places you spend your time can affect your energy, but once you become aware, you'll be able to make changes immediately!

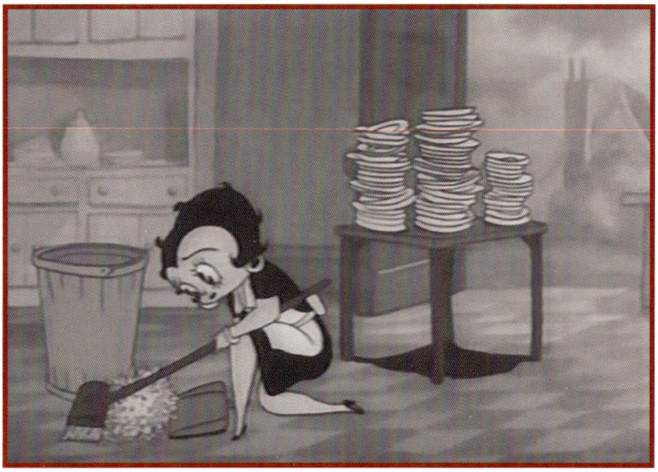

Whether it's your office, bedroom, or entire home, you'll notice a big difference when you take the stuff in there that's draining you and give it the boot! You can begin reducing negative energy and adding more positive vibes to your spaces by clearing clutter first. Clutter is a big creator of negative vibes.

Once you've tackled the clutter, including old papers and magazines, expired medications, stained or torn linens, broken picture frames, old restaurant take-out menus, and other random junk, take a look at the space and get rid of anything else that doesn't serve an important purpose or make you happy in some way. Finally, see if there's a way to bring a bit more natural light to the space if needed. Every space can benefit from an abundance of natural light. If there's not enough natural light coming in through the windows, buy yourself some full-spectrum light bulbs online that mimic natural sunlight. They can make a world of difference.

STEERING CLEAR OF NEGATIVE PEOPLE

This is a big one, so it definitely deserves some focused attention. While we all know that it's in our best interest to spend most of our time with people who inspire us and lift us up, and spend less time with people who leave us feeling drained, it can sometimes be hard to put into practice. Finding ways to distance ourselves from those in our lives who are generally negative and draining can be tricky, especially if they're within our circle of loved ones (and this seems to be the case quite often).

While there are some people we know we need to steer clear of all together, there are some negative people (family members, lifelong friends who are like family, etc.) we may not want (or be able) to cut out completely, but just spend less time around. The way to achieve this is by creating healthy boundaries. Remember, you are not obligated to spend an abundance of time with people who drain you.

There are a few good ways to begin creating healthy boundaries without making it a big to-do. You can start by setting your social media feeds (you can un-follow without having to "unfriend" them) so you no longer see their posts. This is a refreshing small change! You also can screen your calls and simply text someone back if they call and leave a message. You can deliberately but subtly reduce the amount of time you spend with them. You don't have to mention it or make a thing of it, just allow the time you spend with any negative people in your life to quietly and naturally diminish in a healthy way.

Sending birthday or holiday cards in the mail is a good (and boundary-friendly) way to let them know you still care even though you don't see or speak to them as often.

All these "invisible" ways of creating space between you and negative people will begin to have a very noticeable positive effect on your life. It also will free up much needed time to focus on and develop relationships with people who are really great for you (and those for whom you're really great as well).

REDUCE YOUR SCREEN TIME

There's no doubt that computers, smartphones, and televisions can greatly enhance our lives and bring many good things. But with all the good, there also are negative effects that result from all this hyper-connectivity. And, more and more research is beginning to show that too much screen time can have seriously negative effects on our mood and our health.

The blue light emitted from screens can affect our brains in negative ways, especially when it comes to sleep. This "bad" light affects the sleep cycles in our brains, causing insomnia and leading to a host of problems as a result. It's hard to be a positive person full of great energy and optimism when you're tired all the time.

A 2014 report from Nielson found that the average adult logs about eleven hours of screen time per day. Whoa! All this screen time has been shown to increase risk of vision problems, weight gain, chronic fatigue, depression, and a host of other issues. In short, too much screen time is a major source of negativity in our lives.

THE PRINCIPLE– Blue Light Can Have a Dark Side

Betty's Inspiration: *Reducing the negative effects of screen time day by day is easy.*

Just Turn It Off. Most devices today have settings where you can simply turn the blue light off. You also have the option of changing your screen to a better quality of light—one that won't stay with you long after your computer is switched off.

Take a Break. Creating positive habits that get you away from your computer screen can make a big difference. Make sure to get up and move at least once an hour. Spend a little more time with friends in the lunch room, by the water cooler, or outdoors for a quick walk and a few deep breaths. Take that cup of coffee away from the computer and enjoy it in another location—and eat your meals in the kitchen or the cafeteria away from your desk and the computer screen.

Go Old School. You don't have to read *everything* online. Try returning to books, magazines, and newspapers for your daily news and entertainment. Pick up the phone and actually *call* the people on your "to do" list. Instead of emails, send a few thoughtful hand-written notes now and then to friends and family. These small steps can lead to big changes.

Invest in a New Pair of Glasses. If your budget can handle it, buy a pair of glasses with *blue tech lenses*. They filter out much of the blue light we're all exposed to every day from our computers, mobile devices, fluorescent overhead lights, and LED light bulbs. These glasses have clear lenses, are very comfortable, and come in prescription form. They make a wonderful addition to anyone's busy workspace, helping us retain a positive and healthy outlook.

EMBRACING POSITIVE AFFIRMATIONS

Most of us have heard of the practice of using affirmations to help get into the right mindset for something, but how many of us actually use them regularly? Words are powerful. In fact, they're some of the most powerful tools we have in life. The words we use and the way we speak about ourselves and our lives can have an incredible impact.

When you really think about it, nearly everything we say—positive or negative—is an affirmation. When making a statement of any kind, you're affirming whatever it is you're speaking about. Something as simple as saying "I'm going to walk the dog" is an affirmation of your intention to walk your pooch, and believe it or not, saying it out loud makes it more likely to be.

With that, think about the positive effect that's possible when you say something kind and empowering about yourself, such as "I am strong and capable of anything I set my mind to." Doesn't just reading those words feel good? Try saying them out loud. Bang! Right?

Affirmations are magnificent and mighty tools to help give you just the boost you need when you need it. A great strategy is to memorize a few favorites that stir good feelings for you and say them out loud to yourself when you need them.

Write them down on pretty pieces of paper and put them where you can see them. And, for even more benefit, try saying them in front of the mirror.

You can look up great lists of positive affirmations online, write some of your own, or use one or more of our Betty Boop–inspired suggestions below.

I am a beautiful sass-symbol!
I say what I mean and mean what I say!
I'm worthy of all the love in the world!
I am fun, fierce, and fabulous!
I am daring, confident, and irresistible!

One thing everyone can agree on is that the world needs more positivity. Create it. Embrace it. Grab onto it wherever you can. It's not just an outlook, it's a way of life.

DID YOU KNOW?
Some of Betty's favorite social causes include women's heart health awareness and animal rescue organizations.

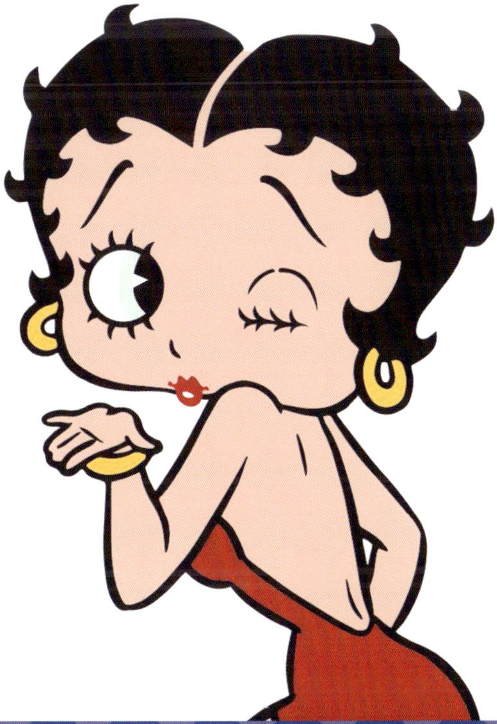

"BE POSITIVE AND THE REST WILL FOLLOW."

Chapter 6

Cultivating Courage

As the storm grew darker, the waves higher and the wind stronger, a frightened Betty Boop and her sidekicks, KoKo the Clown and Bimbo, fought desperately to save themselves and their ship as it was violently tossed in the ocean depths.

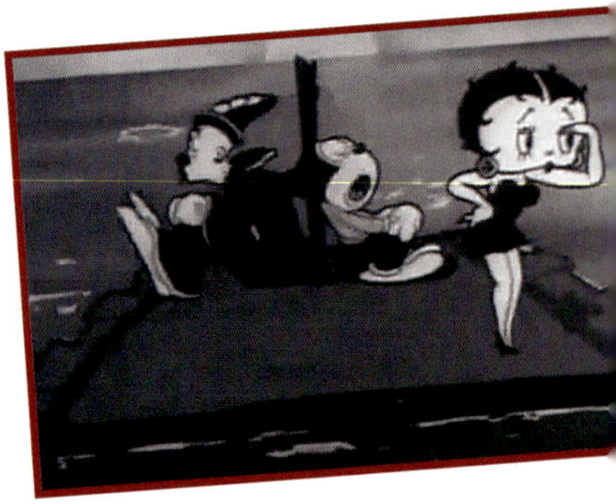

I'm so scared that I can't stand it.
Oh Mama, what can we do?

As she screams through her fears and tears, Betty fights to regain her composure, her confidence, and her courage in the 1932 cartoon *S.O.S.* Originally titled *Swim or Sink,* this is the first time we see Betty terrified of her situation and struggling to survive.

And of course, she perseveres, rises to the occasion, restores her equilibrium, and lives to love another day. Yet, in this cartoon Betty shows us that before we can understand courage, we have to talk about fear.

SO, WHAT EXACTLY IS FEAR? WHAT CAUSES IT? WHERE DOES IT COME FROM?

To answer these questions, we have to resort to a little science.

You see, inside our brain we all have a tiny little almond-shaped area of tissue called the amygdala. As a part of our limbic system, the amygdala is involved in many of our emotions, particularly those related to survival. It's responsible for processing our emotions, including pleasure, anger, and fear. It's also responsible for determining which memories are stored in our brain.

And, this is how it works. When a threat comes along, let's say a spider or a snake, our body reacts quickly to maximize our chances of survival. The amygdala releases stress hormones that sharpen our senses of sight and sound. These hormones also increase our heart rate, which sends blood pulsing through our veins to our muscles so that we can act quickly—and decide to either "stay and fight or take flight."

Fear is defined as an emotional and physical response to danger. And, it's our tiny amygdala that functions as our emergency response unit—historically an absolutely necessary function in the primeval game of survival of the fittest.

Yet, today we humans no longer live in a world where we're constantly threatened by an untamed environment or attacks from wild animals. Rather, our fears today typically revolve around things like uncertainty, rejection, criticism, loss, and failure. And, we're all afraid of something.

You see, fear is a very natural, normal, and common part of human life. For most of us, we will always experience fear in some way of one thing or another. We are not born with courage. Like many other attributes, it's something we have to *cultivate*.

Accordingly, the first step to cultivating courage is to recognize our fear. In order to recognize our fear, we have to be transparent. We have to be open and honest with ourselves. We have to be vulnerable. And remember, *never confuse vulnerability with weakness*.

"... THAT VISIBILITY WHICH MAKES US MOST VULNERABLE IS THAT WHICH ALSO IS THE SOURCE OF OUR GREATEST STRENGTH."
–AUDRE LORDE, WRITER AND CIVIL RIGHTS ACTIVIST

THE PRINCIPLE– Acknowledge Your Fear

Betty's Inspiration: First, face and recognize those things that scare you.

Focus on the Obvious. Are you afraid of being bitten by a dog? Do you fear heights? Are you afraid of flying? Are you afraid of dark basements? Does water scare you? Are you afraid of loud noises or bright lights like thunder and lightning?

When Do You Feel Fear? Is your fear triggered when you're around other people? Do new situations make you fearful? Do you feel fear when you're in public? Are you afraid when you're in a new environment?

Ask Others for Their Opinion. Sometimes other people know us better than we know ourselves. A trusted friend, colleague, or family member can help you recognize the areas of your life that create personal fear.

Review Your Past. Think back to your past. Remember the times you were afraid. Try to remember and identify the events that caused you fear. Fear typically forms a pattern that may repeat itself throughout your life. Understanding your past will help you manage your present.

Write Your Fears Down. Make a list. Write down the fears you recognize—the obvious and the not so obvious ones. Write down what others notice about your fears. Record your memories of past situations in which you felt fear. Writing them down will help you mentally organize your fears. It will move these fears from being buried in the back of your mind to the front of your mind where you can consciously reflect on them.

So, now that we have some understanding of what our fears are, how do we overcome them?

Well, the short answer is we don't. Our goal is not to avoid fear, or step around it, or crawl under it, or jump over it. Our goal is to move through it. Because courage doesn't mean we are without fear. Rather, courage means we see fear, we feel it, we accept it, and we act bravely in spite of it.

"LIFE SHRINKS OR EXPANDS IN PROPORTION TO ONE'S COURAGE."
—ANAÏS NIN, ESSAYIST AND NOVELIST

Cultivating courage is all about learning how to *manage our fears*. And, true courage is a *skill* that can be nurtured, developed, and practiced. Betty has faced many challenges and fears throughout her life. From shipwrecks, to lecherous bosses, to big bullies, to loss, criticism, and embarrassment—and even to ghosts and unworldly specters!

And like most of us, Betty's not a superhero. She's an ordinary girl who, over time, has developed an extraordinary way of looking at the world. Step by step she has become stronger and braver by changing the way she thinks. And, just how did she do this?

Have you ever heard of neuroplasticity? Let's explain it now because this natural phenomenon will be your new best friend.

You see, when we have a particular thought, our brain creates a neural pathway from point A to point B. When this pathway is activated it is brightly lit by thousands of neurons in the brain. When we have the same thought again the brain sees this brightly lit pathway and automatically "goes to the light," sending the same neural impulse down the same pathway. This, of course, results in the same thought and the same reaction.

As this happens over and over again, this pathway becomes deeply engraved in our brain. It becomes a mental rut, not unlike an old rut in a dirt road that has been carved out by hundreds of car tires over many years. And we all know that when we hit a rut in the road, it's very hard to get out of it.

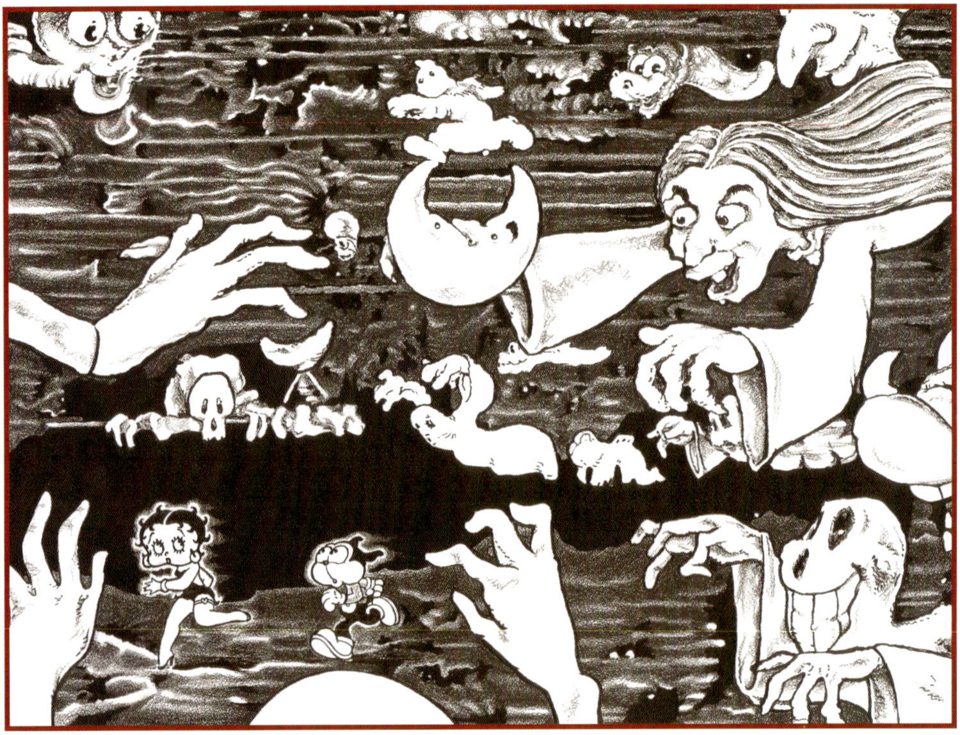

Similarly, when we see a creepy-crawly, a slithering something-or-other, or a wriggling whatnot, our brain remembers the way we reacted the last time. It then jumps to that brightly lit pathway in our brain and sends the same message that we are *scared* and it's time to *scream*!

The good news is that we have the power to change the way our brain works. We have the ability to help our brain reorganize itself and create new neural pathways by feeding it new information. This is neuroplasticity—and it's the cornerstone to managing our fears and cultivating our courage.

THE PRINCIPLE–
Retrain Your Brain

Betty's Inspiration: If you want things to be different, you have to think and act differently.

Learn One New Thing Each Day. Want to know how to say, "thank you" in Italian? Find out! Wondering what that purple flower is in the garden? Look it up! Curious about curry? Pick some up and start cooking! Learning one new thing a day will keep your brain challenged and flexible.

Start Your Day with an Affirmation. We've already discussed the power of positive affirmations. And since we believe you can never have too many, here are a few more for you. "I am capable." "I am strong." "I am brave." "I am not afraid." By doing this, you signal your brain to automatically think in a new and productive way.

Take a Different Route. Stop taking the same route every day. Go three blocks down instead of one. Turn right at the corner instead of left. Travel through a new neighborhood on your way to work. Take the "scenic route" instead of the short cut. Keep it interesting.

Change Up Your Physical Routine. Do you exercise in the morning? Try doing it at night. If you run errands after lunch, do them before instead. Switch up your pattern of working in the yard, taking out the trash, or walking your dog.

Do Your Morning Tasks Differently. If you normally shower first and enjoy coffee after, have your coffee first and then shower. If you return calls and texts before you dress, try getting dressed first and then return your correspondence.

Sound funny? Maybe. Yet, each time you force yourself to think in a new way you are forcing your brain to create new pathways of thought. You are exercising your brain to think in new ways. Before long, in times of stress or fear, your go-to reaction will be one of positive thought and action rather than the same negative thought and action.

And, the next time you encounter that same creepy-crawly, your first instinct may not be to scream. It may be to put a glass over it, take it outside, let it go, and acknowledge that it's probably much more afraid of you than you of it.

Of course, we all know that fear takes many shapes and forms—and no one knows this better than Betty!

Yes, a part of our fear includes anxiety and feelings of repulsion from unwanted small distractions in our environment. It also includes big, large-scale, universal fears that are simply a part of the human condition.

We're all modern women in a modern world. Yet, many of our fears are the same fears that Women like Betty have faced throughout time. And, six of the most common include:

- Rejection
- Uncertainty
- Loss
- Failure
- Ridicule
- Change

Fear can hold us back from achieving our dreams. It can negatively impact our careers, our relationships, and the ways in which we perceive ourselves and our self-worth.

Rejection can keep us from meeting new people. It can prevent us from forming new love interests and friendships. It can scare us away from asking for things that would improve our lives like a raise at work or more help at home. We fear being rejected by individuals and from society in general. This is particularly dangerous because it supports the misconception that our existence is defined and justified only by the acceptance and acknowledgment of others.

Uncertainty keeps us from trying new things. It interferes with our ability to grow and develop. It can frighten us into accepting things as they are rather than acting to make things better. The fear of not knowing what will happen if we attempt to do something new can stifle our progress and evolution. Uncertainty makes it harder for us to explore and understand new things, and makes it easier for us to remain uninspired and closed-minded.

Loss is related to love and fear. When we feel love—for any person, thing, or experience—we naturally fear losing the object of our love. Love brings us happiness, contentment, and fulfilment. No one wants to lose that. There's no doubt that to live, love, and experience life fully is a risky business. Yet, by choosing to live fully in spite of our fear of loss, we create a wondrous opportunity for a life abundant with joy, gratitude, and personal growth.

Failure is a fear that rules over all our actions and decisions. How many times have you decided to do—or not do—something to avoid failing. This fear makes us feel helpless and unable to take charge of any situation or condition. "I'm not good enough." "I won't be able to live with the disappointment if I fail." "Why should I bother trying?"

Ridicule is a fear most of us have experienced since we were children. Once again, it feeds on our need to be accepted by others. It's normal for us to want to belong and feel valued by others. We certainly don't want to be in the "spotlight" where our peers might laugh at us, point fingers at us, or criticize us. This crippling fear once again puts us at the mercy of others where their opinions determine what we feel safe doing and not doing.

Change is a big one—especially if we're happy and content where we are. Yet, change is a natural and organic element of life. Everything in life is always evolving and moving forward. Our fear is triggered by our comparisons of where we are now and where change will take us, which is much like our fear of uncertainty and the unknown. "I'm safe now. Will I be safe if things change?" "I feel loved now. Will I feel loved if things change?" Change is scary because it threatens our stability and may expose our weaknesses.

Betty—sometimes willingly and sometimes not so willingly—has been the poster child of change most of her lifetime. For decades, she has changed her job, her appearance, and her home, never really knowing how things would turn out—yet, always hoping for the best!

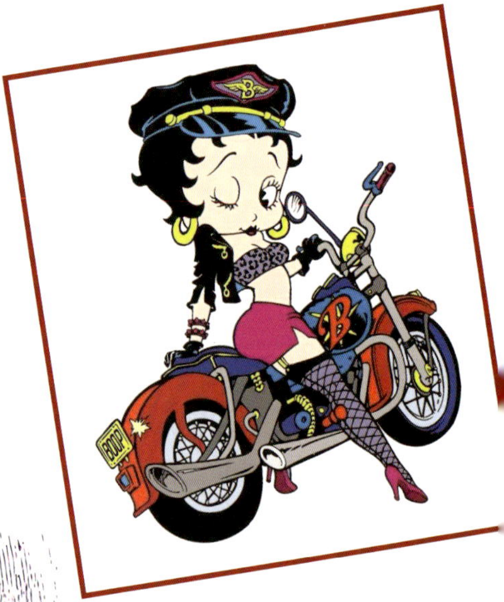

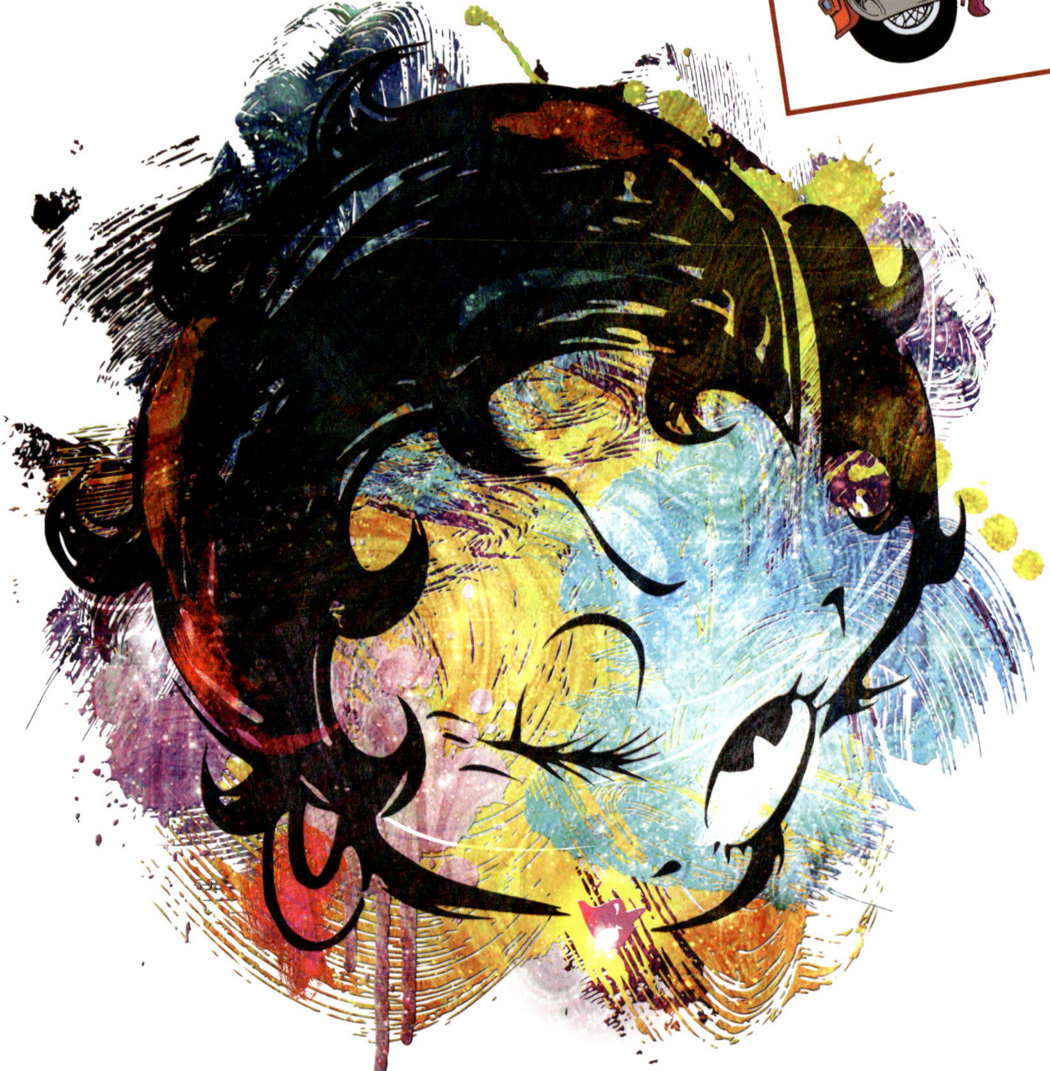

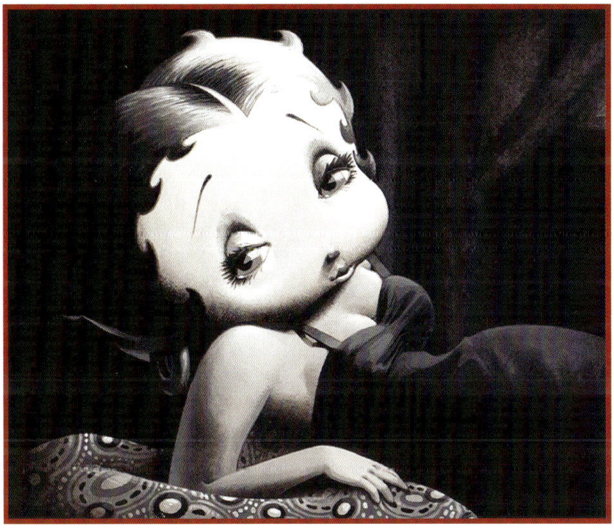

THE PRINCIPLE–
Welcome Change

Betty's Inspiration: Just because it's something new doesn't mean it's something bad.

Don't Panic. Just because change is occurring in your life does not mean you should worry. Remind yourself that every aspect of life changes over time. It's normal and natural. Also, remember that some change is not only necessary to move forward, but also sometimes necessary to ensure a positive outcome. Take a deep breath and relax.

Be Flexible. Change often means that your old ways of doing things may not work anymore. Change demands we see things from new and different perspectives. Listen to others. Read and process new information. Observe the actions of those around you and notice how they may differ from your own. Incorporate new ideas and plans into your everyday goals.

Analyze the Situation. Ask yourself, "What's the worst thing that could happen?" Determine how it may impact your life. Will it destroy your happiness? Will it hurt you or your loved ones? Will it jeopardize your job? Map out every possible outcome. Chances are you'll find that the realistic result of the change you fear will probably never be as bad as your imagination. And, if you can live with the worst that can happen, you can live with everything else.

Practice Acceptance. There are things in life over which we have no control. Change is often one of them. If you face a change you fear, take action to avert it. If your actions fall short, and the change seems inevitable, don't resist. Resistance will only create more stress and anxiety in your life. Instead, accept the change and move forward with a plan of positive action. This will help create a sense of self-empowerment over the situation.

Reflect on Your Past. Think about the ways in which your life has changed over the last ten years. Are you in a better place now because of those changes? Did you learn important lessons from those changes? How have those changes made you a better person? How much of the happiness you now enjoy is the result of those changes? Focus on the positive results of those changes to remind yourself that change can be good.

"THE ONLY WAY THAT WE CAN LIVE,
IS IF WE GROW.
THE ONLY WAY THAT WE CAN GROW,
IS IF WE CHANGE."
—C. JOYBELL C., PHILOSOPHER AND CULTURAL CRITIC

All right then, we know that fear is a natural part of life and we should never expect to be without it. Moreover, there are different kinds of fear. There are *rational* fears and *irrational* fears.

The first include many of those we have already mentioned. Rejection, uncertainty, failure, and change are all rational fears that most of us experience at one time or another. These involve real situations that create anxiety and stress, and may threaten our lives in a significant way.

And ladies, our Betty has confronted many of them. In the 1934 cartoon classic *She Wronged Him Right*, Betty not only faces eviction and the loss of her home, she also has to fight off the villainous advances of an unscrupulous banker.

Things have gone from bad to worse.
No more sugar for my tea.
No more pretty things to wear.
No more ribbons in my hair.

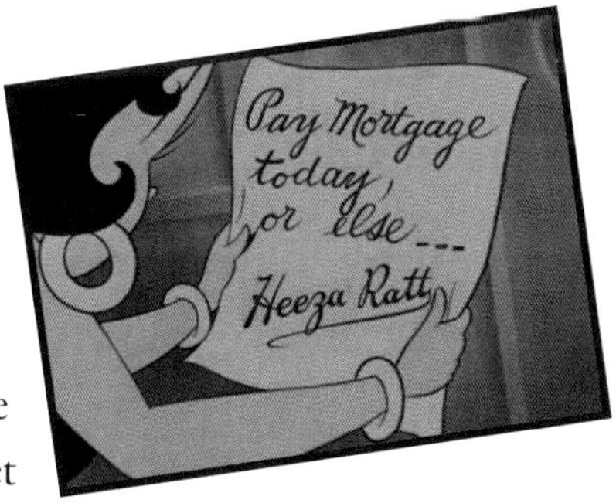

On the other hand, we have *irrational* fears like clowns, the dark, toilet seats, halfway open closet doors, or closed shower curtains.

Chances are the clowns in your life aren't really there to harm you. There probably are no dangers in the basement just because it's dark. It's doubtful you'll catch a life-threatening disease from that toilet seat. And, it's unlikely there's a mass murderer hiding in your closet or behind the shower curtain.

Yet, all fear is controlled by the same tiny almond-shaped amygdala in our brain. There is a science behind fear and there is a science behind courage.

THE COURAGE CENTER

Recently, scientists have discovered that courage is controlled by an area of our brain called the—get ready—*subgenual anterior cingulate cortex*. But we'll call it the *sgACC* for short.

Like the amygdala, the sgACC is a part of the brain's limbic system, which is involved with the functioning of our emotions, including stress, anxiety, and yes, fear. Yet, it's also the driving force behind our courageous acts.

In a wonderful study published in the journal *Neuron*, volunteers were divided into two groups. One group was exposed to a toy teddy bear. The other was exposed to—what else—a live snake. Both groups were told to either move closer to or farther away from these objects.

Needless to say, the group who were given the teddy bear had no trouble moving closer to the object. After all, who's afraid of a cuddly, cute, stuffed toy bear?

The group exposed to the scary snake, on the other hand, reacted differently. As expected, most of them moved farther away from the snake. A few, however, moved closer to the snake.

And, here's what happened! There was no change in the brains of the teddy bear group. Their *Courage Center*, the sgACC, remained inactive. Not a surprise, because the volunteers in this group were not required to be brave. They did not need to activate their Courage Center.

Now, let's look at the volunteers who were given a snake to observe and moved away from it. Not only was their Courage Center *not* activated, their Fear Center in the amygdala *was* activated. Giving in to their fear actually reinforced their particular fear of snakes and strengthened their Fear Center. This means that the next time these people see a snake, they are much more likely to "run away" from it and it will be much harder for them to be brave.

Yet, the group who were exposed to the snake and chose to move even closer to it showed a significant increase in the activity of their Courage Center. It lit up like fireworks! By acknowledging their fear and acting bravely anyway, these volunteers strengthened their Courage Center.

Not only that, but when these volunteers faced their fear and activated their Courage Center, their sgACC automatically shut down the Fear Center in their amygdala. In other words, their courage overshadowed their fear. And, here's our take-away from this study: *Every time we chose to be brave in the face of our fear, we*

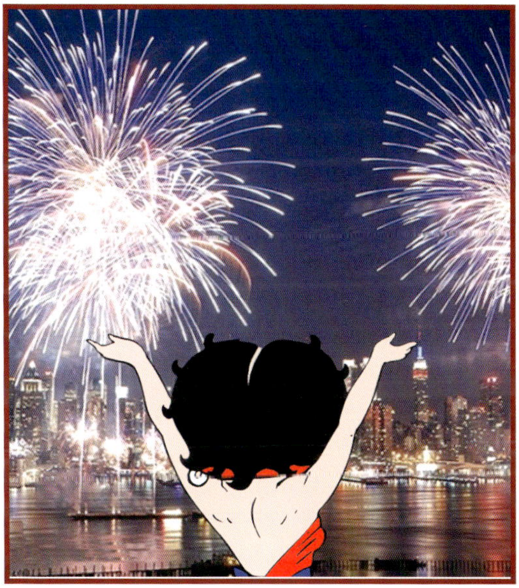

activate our Courage Center. And, every time we activate our Courage Center, it becomes stronger.

It's just like exercising any other muscle in our body. The more we exercise our Courage Muscle, the stronger it becomes. The stronger that muscle becomes, the more our Courage Center is activated. And the more that center is activated, the braver we become. *How cool is that?*

Ever wonder what makes firefighters or doctors or soldiers so brave? Why is it some people seem to have more courage than the rest of us? How come Betty Boop always seems to have the situation—no matter how dire it might be—under control?

The answer, women of the world, is *practice*. We may not feel courageous now, but with a little practice we can all become braver than we are.

"SPEAK YOUR MIND, EVEN IF YOUR VOICE SHAKES."

–MAGGIE KUHN, SOCIAL ACTIVIST AND FOUNDER OF THE GRAY PANTHERS

THE PRINCIPLE–
Exercise Your Way to Courage

Betty's Inspiration: The place you start never has to be the place you stay.

Before We Can Act, We Have to Think. So, let's think thoughts that support our courage and inhibit our fear. Practice visualization. See the fear in your mind. See yourself coming into contact with that fear. Then see yourself passing through that fear to the other side. Every time you do this, you are training your mind to move through fear rather than to avoid it.

Adopt Practices That Help Reduce Stress and Anxiety. Daily physical and mental exercise will help reduce both. Spend a few minutes every day doing some physical exercise. Practice meditation sitting quietly with your eyes closed. Breathe deeply. These techniques help relax our nervous system and reduce the mental noise that inhibit our Courage Center.

Think Positively. Sadness and depression also feed our fear and make it difficult for us to act bravely. Think about the times in your past when you did something brave. Think about how good that made you feel. Think about all the positive outcomes that are possible when you act with courage. Thinking positive thoughts boosts our brain's "feel good" chemicals serotonin and dopamine. These, in turn, help prevent our brain from falling back into the mental "fear rut" while also helping it create new mental pathways and see new possibilities.

Make Your Fears Your Friends. Not every fear is your enemy. For instance, facing one fear may help you better understand something that occurred in your past. Facing another fear may help you learn a new skill like swimming or horseback riding. Facing fear and acting with courage can be a wonderful opportunity to better understand yourself and become a more well-rounded person.

Expose Yourself to Scary Situations. Make a diary of the things that scare you the most. If public speaking is on your list, find every opportunity to speak in front of others. If you're afraid of dogs, volunteer at an animal shelter. Every time you face a fear and act courageously, that fear will be minimized and its hold on you will become weaker.

"DO ONE THING EVERY DAY THAT SCARES YOU."
—ELEANOR ROOSEVELT, FIRST LADY, POLITICAL FIGURE, AND ACTIVIST

LIKE FEAR, THERE ARE DIFFERENT TYPES OF COURAGE

Let's take Betty, for example. We've already mentioned her harrowing experience in 1932 when her ship was sinking in the ocean. This kind of situation requires the type of courage most of us think of first when we think about being brave.

Yet, in the 1936 classic cartoon *Be Human*, Betty confronts a bully who spends his days abusing animals and laughing as the animals cry and cower. Overcoming and dealing with this kind of situation requires a different type of courage.

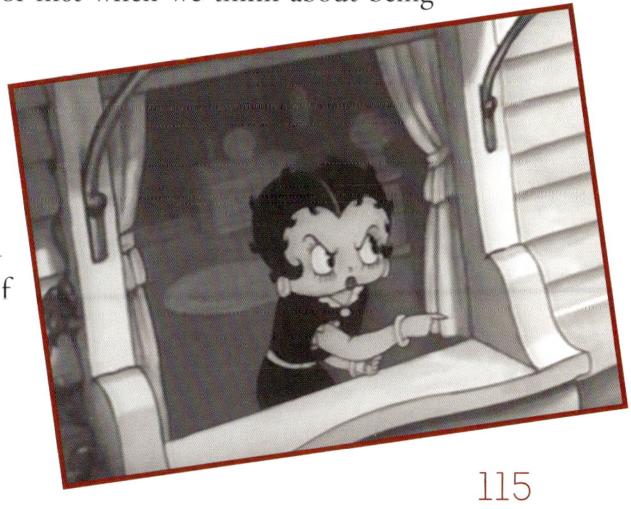

And, six of the most common types of courage include:

- Physical
- Social
- Intellectual
- Spiritual
- Emotional
- Moral

The first, *physical courage*, is the type Betty faced in the middle of the ocean when her ship was sinking in 1932. This involves being brave when faced with the risk of bodily harm or death. Courage here requires us to be aware of frightening situations and resilient at the same time. It involves exercising physical strength and stamina and often disregarding our own safety or pain.

The second, *social courage*, is the type Betty faced above in *Be Human* when she found herself in a situation she knew was wrong. Long before animal cruelty was a crime, Betty recognized this social injustice and found a way to stop the abuse and get even with the abuser. Acting courageous in these situations involves the risk of social exclusion or rejection. It requires us to become leaders even if we end up alone with no support from others.

Intellectual courage challenges us to try new things, engage new ideas, and question our thinking. It forces us to confront confusing or difficult concepts with which we are not familiar. It forces us to step out of our comfort zone and embrace ideological change. It forces us to take new paths in our thoughts and actions and to accept the risk of making mistakes.

Spiritual courage involves facing deeper issues than those we deal with on a daily basis. Why am I here? What is my purpose in life? What happens when I die? Asking these profound existential questions can be scary. As human beings, we want definitive answers to our questions about life. When we ask this type of question, however, we must accept the fact that we are unlikely to find definitive answers. This type of courage requires us to accept the unknown and be open to the mysteries of life.

Emotional courage is displayed when we recognize our faults, our limitations, our weaknesses, and still totally accept ourselves despite them. This courage requires us to feel and act without expecting anything in return. It asks us to give of ourselves and our hearts even in the face of rejection. Rather than suppressing, ignoring, or denying our emotions, this courage asks us to embrace them—as flawed as they may be. In doing so, we position ourselves to accurately assess our experiences and avoid faulty decision-making.

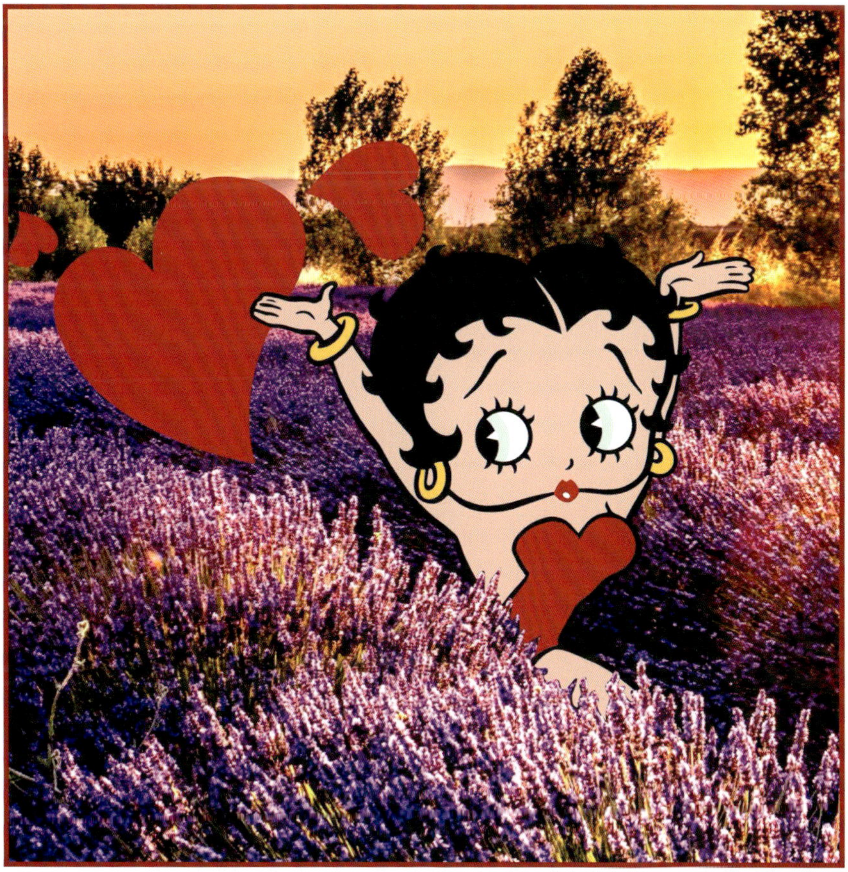

Moral courage means doing the right thing even at the risk of losing security, social status, or favor with others. This courage requires that we rise above the hatred, apathy, and violence of the world around us. It means listening to that little voice that tells us what we should do. We are guided by our conscience, not the pressures of the outside world.

THE LOVE FACTOR

Now, here's the really cool thing about the human condition and the way our nervous system works. We can't be in a state of fear and a state of love at the same time. This means the more we cultivate peace of mind, physical ease, and comfort, the less we feel fear. And, the less we feel fear the more likely we are to be courageous.

Let's analyze Betty. She faces fear because *she feels passionate* about something, she loves someone or something, she is trying to right a wrong. She is dedicated to something beyond her own feelings or desires. Her courage center is triggered by something bigger than her own feelings—including her feelings of fear.

"PASSION IS AND SHOULD ALWAYS BE THE HEART OF COURAGE."
–MIDORI KOMATSU, ACTRESS AND DANCER

In other words, when Betty is connected to her Love Center, her personal feelings of anger and fear are overshadowed by her feelings of love and commitment.

As we discussed in chapter 2, we know how important love is, so let's touch on it as it relates to courage. When our Love Center is activated our brain produces more of those wonderful endorphins serotonin and dopamine. Our love hormone, oxytocin, increases and we begin to feel great! And, in this state of well-being and safety, it's easier for Betty—and all of us—to act courageously.

THE PRINCIPLE–
Connect to Love

Betty's Inspiration: Love is the foundation that fights Fear and opens the door to Courage.

Enjoy Mother Nature. Get outside. Breathe fresh air. Pick some flowers. Plant a tree. Take a walk. Hike in the hills. Go jump in a lake. Literally.

Listen to Your Favorite Music. This is the perfect antidote to stress and anxiety. It relaxes our nervous system. It eases mental and physical pain, discomfort, and plain old grumpiness. As the saying goes, "Music soothes the savage breast."

Lend a Helping Hand. Helping another who is less fortunate than yourself is a great way to fight fear and depression. The act of aiding others forces us to move away from our own problems and focus on the needs of others.

Remember to Practice Gratitude. Remember this discussion? Gratitude will always connect us to love. Life will never be perfect. There will always be things that anger us, annoy us, and aggravate us. Yet, focusing on the good things in our life will change our outlook and allow us to feel better about ourselves and the world around us.

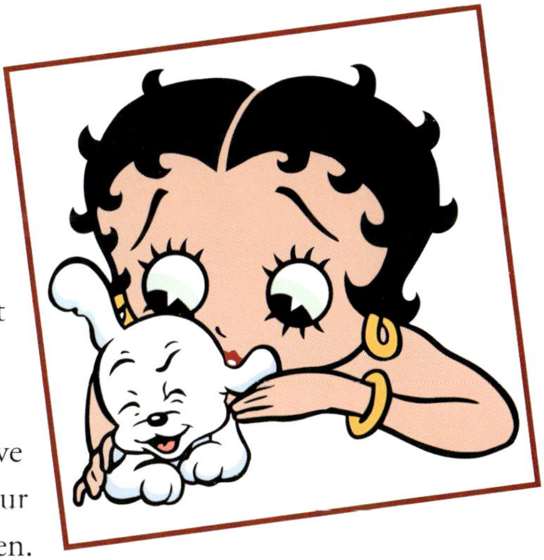

Spend Time with Loved Ones. Nothing inspires love like love. Hold your loved ones close. Play with your dog. Tell someone you love them. Hug your children. Just eight hugs a day will increase our love-ly oxytocin, making for a happier you and a better world.

We'll never be without fear. It's part of life in an ever-changing and uncertain world. But, little by little, we can cultivate courage—lasting courage that doesn't have to be loud, powerful, or explosive to be effective. Because, courage in every form, no matter how small or quiet, is courage. Plain and simple. And, just like Betty, we can become a little braver each day, one small step at a time.

"COURAGE DOESN'T ALWAYS ROAR. SOMETIMES COURAGE IS THE LITTLE VOICE AT THE END OF THE DAY THAT SAYS I'LL TRY AGAIN TOMORROW."
–MARY ANNE RADMACHER, WRITER AND ARTIST

DID YOU KNOW?
Betty Boop appeared in more than 100 cartoons over her career and was nominated for an Oscar in the 1938 classic *Riding the Rails*.

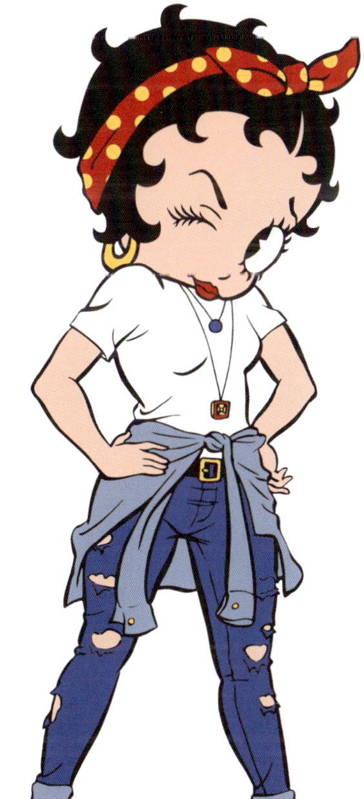

"A FEAR
FACED IS A
FEAR ERASED."

Chapter 7

Confidence: The Must-Have Accessory

Confidence truly is an amazing, magical thing. When you are confident, people see you as more charismatic, more able, more together, and even more fun. The best part is that when you feel confident, you see *yourself* as those things too! That's why building solid self-confidence is so important to feeling empowered and living our best life. Unfortunately, a variety of life circumstances from childhood all the way through our adult years can sometimes chip away at our self-confidence and self-esteem.

The good news is that with some dedication and practice, we can all build more confidence and greater self-esteem. Learning to embrace and love all the things that make us who we are so we can have a solid foundation of self-confidence is what this chapter is all about. Get ready to celebrate and believe in your fabulous self more than ever!

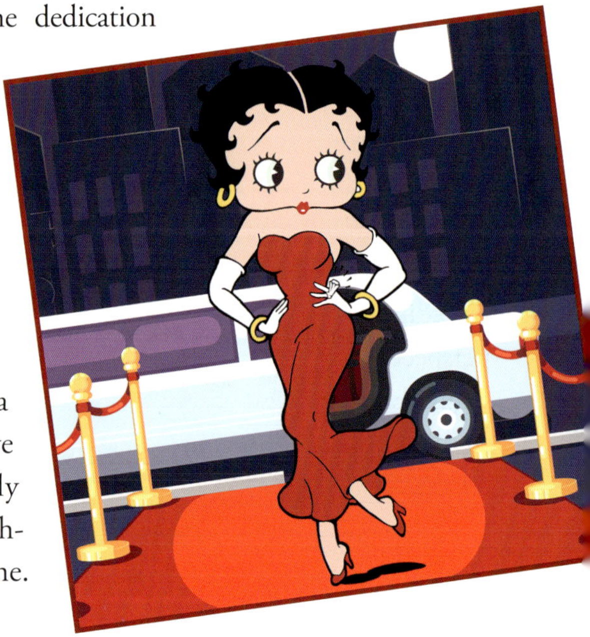

With social media now such a significant part of our lives, we live in a world where we are constantly tempted to compare ourselves to others and the images they portray online.

Comparison (usually to photos online that are totally filtered or to posts that include only the good stuff) can lead us to being hard on ourselves for a variety of unnecessary reasons. We can be critical of ourselves for not having the perfect house, the perfect clothes, the perfect hair, the perfect . . . whatever. The problem is that we're comparing ourselves to carefully edited, unrealistic illusions without even having the whole story.

In the 1937 cartoon *Ding Dong Doggie*, Betty's pup Pudgy sees a Dalmatian and decides that he too wants to have spots and ride on a neat fire truck! He even goes as far as to paint spots on his coat. When he hears the fire truck roaring down the street, Pudgy tags along with his new Dalmatian friend to help fight a fire and quickly learns the hard way that fire-fighting is not what he's meant to do at all! In the end, he discovers that he's happy being who he is and is overjoyed to get back home after his rough day—even when Betty is angry with him for having gone missing all day.

All the (false) perfection and unrealistic images portrayed online—and in celebrity pop-culture magazines, too—can lead to telling ourselves untrue stories about who we are and what we should be doing in the world in comparison to everyone else. It's the modern-day version of keeping up with the Joneses.

Being bombarded with so many unrealistic images, for some of us, also can bring on that awful, familiar feeling of "not enough." It's very important to know one big, important truth with absolute certainty—that *you* are *always* enough! No matter what, *we* are all always *enough*.

The actual truth is we're all doing our best, we've all had major setbacks in life, and we all have imperfections that are part of making us the unique and incredible people we are. And, when we closely examine our lives with a fresh perspective, we can see that there are truly wonderful things worth celebrating regularly! All the things that make you uniquely you are the things that make you so incredibly special. You deserve to be celebrated just as you are!

RADICAL SELF-CONFIDENCE

With all we're exposed to daily in today's world, it's as important as ever to develop a radical, bullet-proof sense of self-confidence. It's like a suit of armor

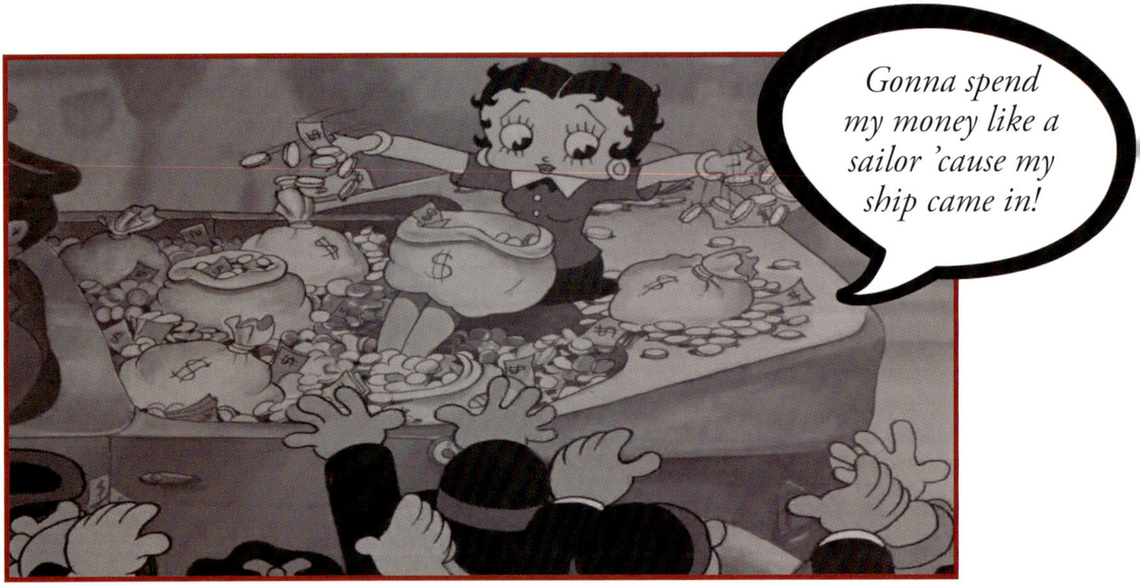

that will be there to aid and protect you through all your journeys, both harrowing and wonderful.

We all—every single one of us—have valuable contributions to offer the world. Realizing our own value is an important, positive part of our self-worth. Betty Boop is a great example of a woman who has always embodied this idea.

In the 1934 cartoon *When My Ship Comes In,* Betty shows confidence in herself and in her decisions as she wins a large sum of money on a horse race, and then decides to spend it on others instead of herself. She believes in her vision and how it might help her community overcome the Great Depression.

Confidence doesn't literally mean spending your money like a sailor, of course. It just means trusting your ideas and believing in your vision, as well as believing in your amazing self. We're all guilty of not giving ourselves enough credit when we deserve it. We tend to overlook our own greatness when truthfully we should always be looking for (and celebrating!) the greatness within us. Learning to recognize just how strong, capable, and fabulous we actually are is a sure way to building more confidence. But this is often easier said than done, right? Fortunately, there are a number of helpful ways to build upon this that can deliver great results. Let's talk about a few tips for building radical self-confidence. Sound good?

THE PRINCIPLE–
Believe in You

Betty's Inspiration: Every day is a good day to celebrate being you!

Act as If. What does this mean? Well, confident people *act as if* they belong or as if they know what they're doing in any situation—even when they feel like they don't. They are confident enough to consciously overcome any limiting beliefs they may have about a situation. At the same time, they're not afraid to ask for help or directions if they need it, but they do so in a self-assured way with a smile. Hold your head up, proceed with purpose (just like Betty does), and act as if. Not only will everyone around you see your confidence, you'll *feel* more confident which will help you navigate whatever it is in front of you.

Celebrate Your Uniqueness. Take a few moments now and then to remember how special you truly are! There is nobody else in the world like you. There are other people who may say similar things, or do similar things, but there is absolutely no one who will say or do them in exactly the way you will! So, the next time you're tempted to stay quiet because you think someone else has already said what's on your mind, remember, there is no one who has said it in the same way you can! The world needs your uniqueness!

Have a Party for One. You don't need a special occasion to celebrate—you *are* the special occasion! Every now and then when the mood strikes, for no reason whatsoever, pour yourself a glass of champagne or cup of flavorful herbal tea, make yourself your favorite meal, bake a special cake, and simply celebrate being you!

Give Yourself More Credit. Truly! Take a couple of minutes to think about some of your big accomplishments, what a good friend/family member you are to others in your life, and a few other things you know you're good at. It's so easy to recognize these things in others, but unfortunately it's even easier to take our own outstanding qualities for granted. Really think on this one. Close your eyes and give yourself all the credit you know you're due. Say to yourself, "You are fun, fierce, and fabulous!" Make a practice of doing this regularly.

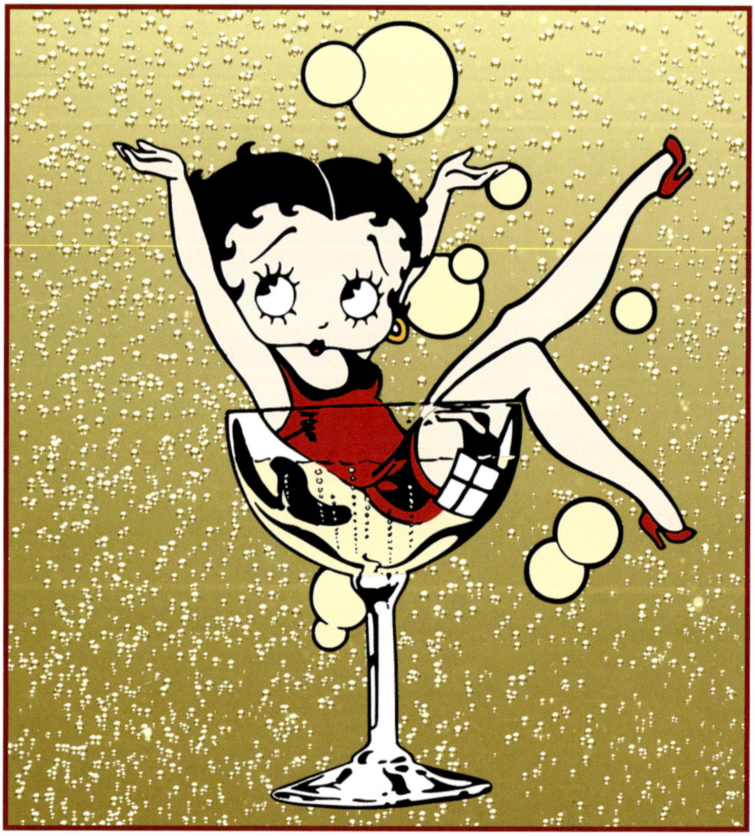

CHANGE THE STORIES YOU TELL YOURSELF

> "BABY, YOU'RE A FIREWORK!"
>
> —KATY PERRY, POP STAR AND ACTIVIST

Part of giving ourselves proper credit where more credit is due involves being willing to re-create the stories we tell ourselves about various events that have occurred. For example, let's say you were on the swim team in high school and you have a sad memory about "messing up" an important race. But, when you take a fresh look back at the situation, you might see that when you woke up with a cold that morning, you could have easily stayed home. You could have just not even gone to the meet! But instead, you picked yourself up and went to compete, even though you felt awful. You didn't actually lose that race, if you think about it. You won just by showing up and getting in that pool! Many people would have just stayed home, but you showed up! You deserve balloons and a parade.

See what a difference telling a new version of a story can make for your confidence? It doesn't matter how much time has passed since an event that created a painful memory took place. It's never too late to change the story. Isn't that a great thought? Think of a few memories in your life where you've been hard on yourself and see if there might be a new version of the story in there somewhere. There almost always is, and when you see it, it can create such a wonderful positive change. Sad memories turn into happy ones. Disempowering memories turn into empowering ones!

Moving forward in your life, make it a habit to always see yourself in the best possible light—and tell your future stories in ways that give you the credit you deserve.

BE BOLD ENOUGH TO TRY NEW THINGS

Are you missing out on things in life because you're afraid to try and learn about them? Do you have a little voice in your head that tells you you're not tech-savvy, that you don't want to travel alone, or that you "don't like" sushi (or any other food) even though you've never even tried it? These limiting beliefs may be holding you back from creating the bigger, bolder life you deserve.

This is especially limiting when it comes to avoiding technology because you think you won't "get it." You are more tech-savvy than you think! There are apps and other technological advances out there that can improve your life and make things easier for you if you're willing to give them a chance. No one "ages out" of technology. If a fifth grader can do it, you can too!

For example, Betty and her team have a dear friend who is hard of hearing and well into his seventies! He uses a wonderful app on his phone that helps him understand what people around him are saying. It's such a great tool and is especially useful in loud and chaotic environments like restaurants, parties, and sporting events.

By the way, Betty's own Grampy is a champion of innovation and technology. Over the years Grampy has taken simple household items and from them has created central air conditioning, dishwashers, robotic vacuum cleaners, prostheses for disabled animals, vending machines, and the very first luggage on wheels! And in the 1936 cartoon classic *Grampy's Indoor Outing*, he built an entire indoor carnival replete with musical swings, shooting galleries, and a roller coaster. Grampy was never afraid to jump in the deep end, experiment with and embrace new technology. All it took was a little inventive imagination and confidence in himself!

So, why not challenge yourself right now to try some new technology, or any other thing you've been afraid to try, ASAP. After you go for it, you'll find yourself saying, "That was so easy! I should have tried that a long time ago!"

You have the power and freedom to expand your horizons in so many areas! Is there a trip you've always dreamed of taking, but haven't done because you're afraid of traveling alone? Go for it! Solo travel can be wonderful and soul-expanding! Is there a person you've been wanting to get to know better but you've been too shy to make a call or send that friend request? You can do it! You know that fantastic empowered feeling you get when you take a leap and do something outside of your comfort zone? What if you could have that wonderful feeling more often? Trying new things (and things you're afraid of) will bring it!

DISSOLVING SELF-DOUBT

Self-doubt is like an epidemic! It can hold us back, influence the choices we make, and contribute to keeping us small. It affects us all from time to time, but those with the greatest self-confidence are affected the least. So, what are some of the best ways we can reduce self-doubt and be more confident when it comes to making choices or even when walking into a room?

One way we can begin to dissolve self-doubt is to learn to catch ourselves when it starts creeping in. This can happen in a variety of situations, but we're especially prone to this when it comes to making choices. We all know what self-doubt feels like. It shows up as negative self-talk or as a nagging, negative feeling in the back of your mind. If you train yourself to notice when these feelings start to bubble up, they can be quickly reduced by simply changing the words you're saying to yourself, and by actively choosing to remember how capable you really are! This can stop the self-doubter within you cold, and inspire new, positive feelings about the situation.

Another effective tool for dissolving self-doubt is to talk to positive-minded friends about your feelings. Believe it or not, pep talks do actually work and we can all benefit from a good one now and then. Let them tell you how confident they are in you, and really listen to each word. Hearing how much others believe in you will remind you that you're absolutely worth believing in.

If you're up for starting a small, life-changing little habit that will boost confidence and good feelings, as well as help abolish self-doubt, try starting a journal celebrating yourself. Get yourself a pretty journal (there are some adorable Betty Boop ones available!) and at the end of each day, write at least one win that you had that day, or one thing you did that was pretty great. It can be the smallest thing . . . it all counts! You also can use this journal to write down things you're grateful for. When you dedicate yourself to this practice each day, you'll find that you'll begin to focus much more on your wins, your blessings, and on giving yourself credit when you deserve it. Plus, it's fun to flip through it to be reminded how amazing you are any time you need a confidence boost!

HAVING CONFIDENCE IN YOUR CHOICES

Let's cover choices. This is one of the areas in life where self-doubt can really show up big. Important choices like taking a new job or small choices like which cereal to buy at the grocery store, it doesn't matter. Self-doubt can creep in and sneak up on us at any time. Perhaps you're a bit haunted by choices you made in the past that didn't turn out so great. Or, maybe you're afraid of making a mistake. It's important to know you're not alone here. These are things that affect everyone. So, the key is to focus on the good and acknowledge your previous successes while forgiving yourself for any mistakes of the past. After all, you learned from those experiences and you've come a long way since then! All your life experiences—great and not so great—are exactly what empower you with the understanding and wisdom to make good choices today.

Remember the Things You're Afraid of are Very Unlikely

Having more confidence in your choices and decisions can mean getting a handle on those things you fear. When faced with a choice, our minds naturally tend to run through all the terrible things that might happen as a result. The fact is our minds can tend to make things out to be so much worse than they actually would be in the (very small) chance they actually occur. Taking a step back and allowing yourself to have a realistic look at the big picture is a powerful habit to adopt.

Remember when we were discussing courage and our fear of change? We all tend to focus on the potential negative outcomes of a situation instead of allowing ourselves to focus on the possible positive outcomes. Now, this is not to say that you shouldn't weigh possible consequences of a decision before you make it, it's just to say don't let yourself get stuck there. Allow yourself to examine all the possibilities and if this choice seems like one you want to go after, empower yourself by focusing on your desired positive outcome. This is what will propel you forward and give you the confidence you need to take the leap.

Know That Failures Are Temporary

Failure is nothing to be afraid of. Yes, sometimes it can feel like a real bummer when it happens. But in truth, it is a necessary part of the path to success! The lessons that can come from it are often invaluable, and sometimes it's even a blessing because you come to realize it was pushing you in the direction you were meant to be headed in the first place. Knowing this—and trusting in whatever the outcome of a choice may be—will make you much less afraid of failure, and more excited about moving forward with any decisions you make.

Brushing off the Naysayers

In order to build a solid foundation for impenetrable self-confidence, we must become quite good at brushing off the naysayers. There will always be those who will express doubt or misguided concern about what you're up to. The key is to clearly recognize the difference between genuine, valid concern from a caring ally and the well-meaning doubt someone might express because of their own fear of change or failure (or sometimes simply because it's their nature to be a negative nelly!).

Most of us have at least one person in our life that always seems to try to talk us out of bold choices or big changes. It might be a friend or relative who is genuinely goodhearted, so the negativity they express can throw us off course if we let it because these are the people we love and trust. Or, sadly, it may just be a negative person who is envious of your courage and is looking to hinder your success.

Recognizing that our choices will never please everyone can be incredibly freeing as well as emboldening. Give yourself permission to disappoint a few people! Know that this is part of creating your best life and making the choices that are right for *you*. After all, only you can know what your heart really wants.

"NOTHING HAS TRANSFORMED MY LIFE MORE THAN REALIZING THAT IT'S A WASTE OF TIME TO EVALUATE MY WORTHINESS BY WEIGHING THE REACTION OF THE PEOPLE IN THE STANDS."
—BRENE BROWN, RESEARCH PROFESSOR AND AUTHOR

BOOSTING YOUR SELF-ESTEEM

Although self-confidence and self-esteem are two different things, they definitely go hand-in-hand. In order to have solid self-confidence, a strong sense of self-esteem is a must. Some people have a natural, healthy sense of self-esteem, and some may be in need of some helpful nurturing to re-build self-esteem after life's circumstances have diminished it. One thing's for sure: we can all use some beneficial tools and concepts to fortify our self-esteem, whether the boost we're in need of is small or large.

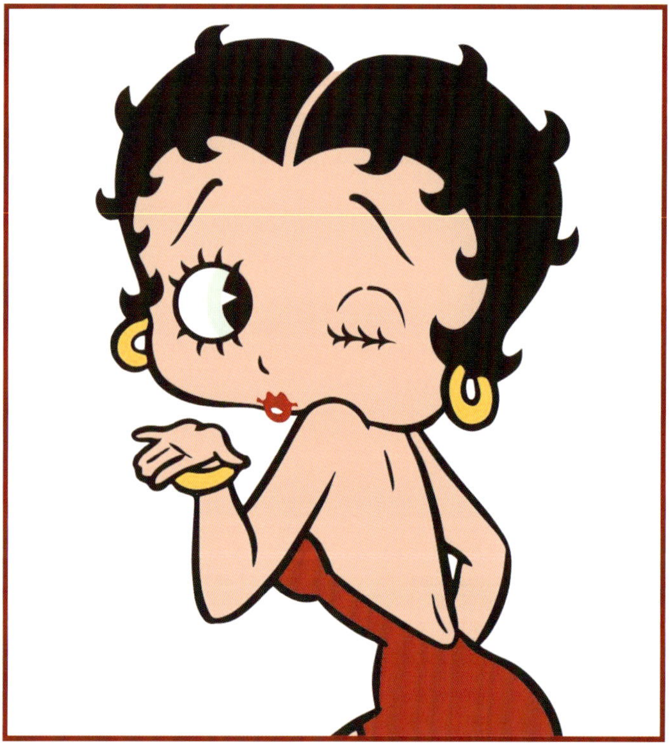

THE PRINCIPLE– You Deserve the Best in Life

Betty's Inspiration: You are worthy of love and other wonderful things.

Know Your Worth. Your opinions matter. Your desires matter. *You matter*. Become extra bold when it comes to standing up for yourself and knowing that you are of equal value to all other humans. It's easy to buy into the notion that someone else's opinion matters more, or that another person's career, hobby, or goals are more important. You are as worthy and deserving of love, respect, and success as any other person.

Believe You Deserve the Best. There are two key parts to having the best life has to offer, and the first (and most important) part is believing you *deserve* it. You definitely do, just for being you! The second part is knowing that we get out of life what we put into it, so knowing we deserve the best can be inspiration for offering the best version of ourselves to the world.

See How Fabulous Life Already Is. Taking a good look at all the wonderful things you currently have in your life, realizing how fabulous life *already* is, and recognizing that you deserve these good things is a big part of the path to attracting even *more* fantastic things.

Value Your Time. A powerful element of confidence is knowing that our own time is as valuable as anyone else's. And, protecting our time as though it was our most valuable commodity (spoiler alert: it is!) is part of creating our best life. It's not okay for someone to keep you waiting long when you had an appointment, or to take your time for granted in any way. Being confident enough to set healthy boundaries when it comes to your time can be truly life-changing! And in return, by similarly valuing the time of others you'll create good vibes across the board!

BETTY'S #1 TIP FOR SELF-CONFIDENCE

If Betty could offer just one big tip for building self-confidence and self-esteem, it would definitely be to *get to know yourself and your strengths even better than you already do*! When you are crystal clear about your strengths and you have a list in your mind of things you like about yourself, you see yourself and the world through a more joyful, more confident lens.

Not quite sure what your greatest strengths are? Take a survey! Ask those who know and love you what they think your greatest strengths are. They'll be honest and you might even be pleasantly surprised!

As you know by now, Betty is a big believer in making lists. In fact, Betty and her friends don't think you can ever have enough lists! So, when it comes to acknowledging the things you like about yourself, why not try this? Take a journal or pretty piece of paper and write down a minimum of ten things you really like about yourself. Sense of humor? A good cook? A green thumb? Your caring and kind soul? Write them all down and keep the list handy in a place where you'll see it regularly. Writing them down will help you remember them, and remembering them will do wonders for boosting confidence. It's always a feel-good thing to remember those things that make you uniquely likeable and loveable!

BE WILLING TO LEAP

A healthy foundation of confidence can lead us to taking leaps in life that can get us far. But, taking those leaps also can require willingness to go outside our safe zone for a bit, as well as something else we talk about in this book—courage! The good news is that the more you take leaps (yes, small leaps count!), the easier it will become!

Betty Boop has always believed in her abilities, even if she may not always be 100 percent sure what she's getting into. This, of course, has brought her to many fantastic and hilarious adventures! In the fun 1935 cartoon *Judge for a Day*, Betty is a court reporter who knows in her heart that she could make a difference and make the world a better place if she could just be the judge. Haven't we all felt that way at one time or another?!

This town is full of pests! Make me judge for a day and I'll get a hold of all of these pests and teach them a lesson!

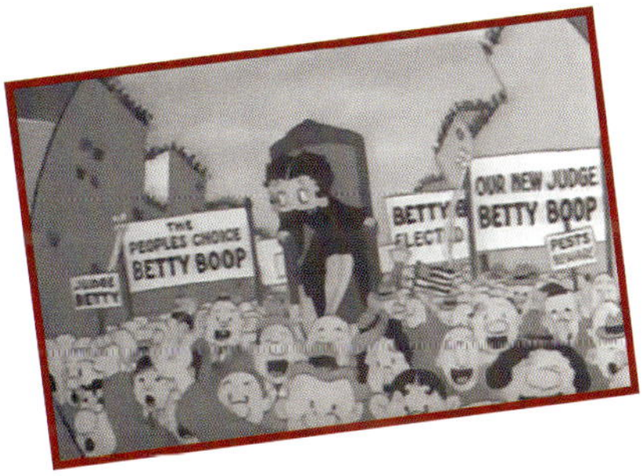

Knowing herself and being confident in her abilities, Betty does get the chance to become judge for a day, deftly handling herself and doling out justice just where it was needed! The townspeople are so happy with what she accomplishes that they celebrate her with a parade. All because she was willing to take a leap!

You are capable of so much more than you realize! Believe in yourself and nurture your confidence on a regular basis and see what an amazing difference it really can make!

"IT'S CONFIDENCE IN OUR BODIES, MINDS, AND SPIRITS THAT ALLOWS US TO KEEP LOOKING FOR NEW ADVENTURES."
–OPRAH WINFREY, TELEVISION PERSONALITY, ACTRESS, AND AUTHOR

DID YOU KNOW?

Margie Hines was the first voice-actor to play Betty Boop, although Mae Questel, who began voicing Betty in 1931, was Betty's most notable and enduring voice.

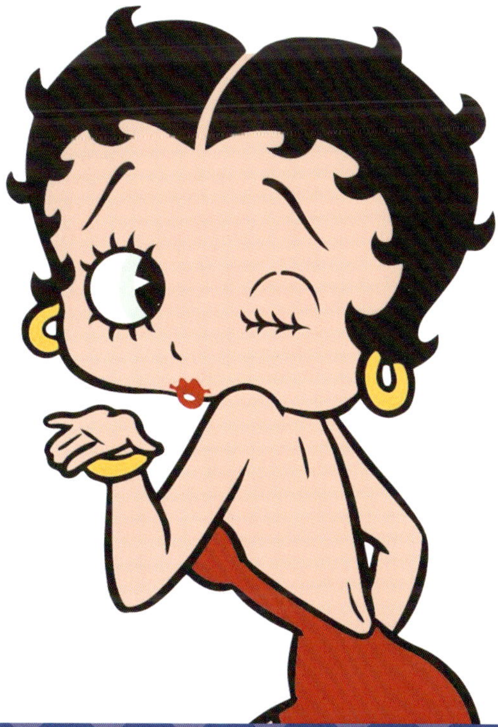

"BELIEVE IN
YOURSELF
A LITTLE
MORE."

Chapter 8

Humor Makes the World Go 'Round

The year is 1937. The place is the Hi-De-Ho-Tel. And, Betty Boop and her beloved Grampy are in charge of all the tired travelers, the restaurant, and the grounds of this forty-room and two-bath establishment. What could possibly go wrong?

Get somebody quickly, there's a mouse in the house!
Everything is messy, come at once with a broom!
This place is very dusty and I think I'm gonna' sneeze!
It's too noisy! It's too hot! It's too cold!
When is dinner ready and I won't say please!

Betty is bombarded with angry complaints and try as she does, she just can't fix anything or make anyone happy. That is until she and Grampy join forces and decide to laugh and smile their way through all the problems.

This is Betty. We give you service with a smile. Boop-Oop-a-Doop!

Perhaps the most enduring quality of our Betty is her ability to look on the bright side of life, to find a way to smile when things get tough, and to laugh in spite of the troubles she encounters along the way. For nine decades, she has always landed on her feet. And to this day, her sense of humor remains intact.

SO, WHAT'S HER SECRET?

How does she do it? Can we be more like Betty?

The good news here is that all of us have the ability to be more like Betty.

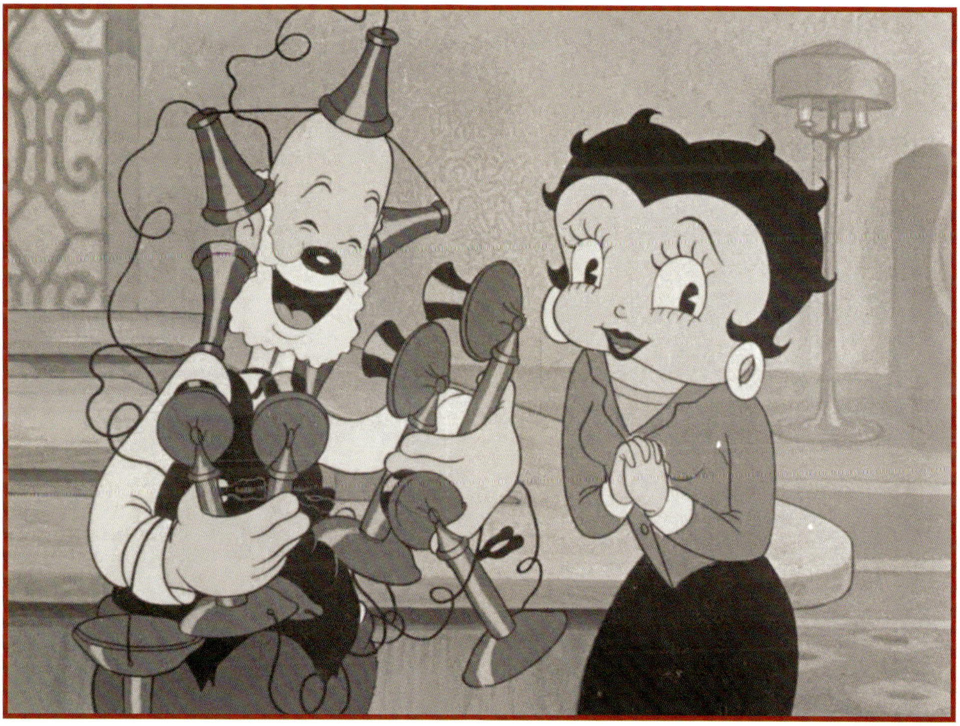

You see, we're all human beings. And, the experience of humor or light-heartedness is innate and inborn in every individual—and even in many of the creatures around us.

But first, let's separate "humor" from the attributes of humor like laughing and smiling. Because they are, after all, different things.

Humor is defined by the fabulous folks at *Merriam-Webster* as "the ability to be amused." This means we're able to laugh at jokes, humorous situations, funny visual cues, and a variety of other potential sources of amusement or light-heartedness.

But there's more to it than that. After all, most of us can exercise humor when faced with something fun or funny. In fact, this ability develops at a very early age. Humans actually begin to react with humor to their surroundings within a few weeks of birth.

Yet, humor also encompasses the overall ability to appreciate whatever life throws at us. It not only includes our ability to recognize that which is truly funny like the latest "knock-knock" joke, but also those things that are obtuse, out of place, or just plain ridiculous or surprising. And most of all, true humor is a skill that allows us to appreciate the ironies of life and to "see the humor" in life's absurdities.

> "IF YOU COULD CHOOSE ONE CHARACTERISTIC THAT WOULD GET YOU THROUGH LIFE, CHOOSE A SENSE OF HUMOR."
>
> –JENNIFER JONES, ACTRESS

Humor is a tool that prevents us from taking ourselves or the world around us too seriously. It enables us to distance ourselves a bit from the action and to become more of a witness to a situation rather than a participant in the situation. And when this occurs, we become more comfortable when things turn upside down. We become less obsessed with keeping everything normal and proper. We become better at perceiving the bigger picture, the overall patterns, and the idiosyncrasies of an unpredictable world. In short, we become better able to handle all the twists and turns of life, including those of an unfortunate or distressing nature.

So, you see, having a "sense of humor" is not dependent on actually seeing or hearing something fun or funny. Just ask Betty! Throughout her career, she's been faced with loss, pain, toil, and trouble of every kind. Yet, she finds a way to steady herself, get back on her feet, and move forward with conviction and grace. And, no matter what you may face you can do the same!

XOXO

THE PRINCIPLE–
Keep Humor Front and Center

Betty's Inspiration: Don't despair! No matter what happens, you can always land on your feet!

Laugh Every Day. Think of it like brushing your teeth or washing your face. Make a conscious effort to find something each day that makes you laugh. Set aside ten or fifteen minutes to do something amusing. The more you laugh, the more natural it becomes and the less effort you'll have to make.

Don't Take Yourself so Seriously. Learn to laugh at yourself even when life is hard. Know that not every day will go as you plan. Invent a funny story about that tough situation or that embarrassing moment. Try to make up a humorous anecdote that will make others laugh and possibly help them through the same thing.

Surround Yourself with Mementos That Remind You to Lighten Up. Keep pictures close by of you and loved ones having fun. Use a screensaver that makes you laugh. Hang a few funny posters. Keep a silly toy in your car or on your desk.

When Funny Things Do Happen, Write Them Down. Make notes of the uplifting things that occur throughout your day. Think about them often and share them with others—especially when you're feeling blue or grumpy.

TOOLS OF THE TRADE

LAUGHTER

The laugh. It's unifying, it's universal, and it's the most important ice-breaking component of a healthy human sense of humor.

"MY FAMILY HATES MY COOKING SO MUCH THEY BOUGHT ME AN OVEN THAT FLUSHES."
–PHYLLIS DILLER, COMEDIENNE AND AUTHOR

As human beings, laughter is our birthright. It's something we humans have shared, well, probably forever! Did you know that human babies begin to chuckle within the first few weeks of life? Did you know that they laugh out loud within a few months? And, did you know that as adults, we women laugh about seventeen times a day?

Yet after all this time, laughter remains one of the most puzzling of human behaviors. Think about it. When we laugh our mouths open up, strange noises come out that have no meaning like words do, we spit and sometimes cry, our eyes bulge, we gasp for breath, hold our sides, and turn red in the face as our bodies convulse and contort. It's quite odd, really.

Strangely, it's believed that laughter through the ages has been linked to the evolution of the human brain. No kidding! You see, the brain evolved to solve complicated ecological problems related to survival, such as learning to hunt, cook, and use tools. Yet, the brain also evolved to allow humans to cope with the social demands of living in larger groups and tribes.

According to the "social brain" hypothesis, as humans began to bond together, the need to communicate became more urgent. The brain evolved and language developed as individuals searched for a way to establish their new bond with larger groups of individuals.

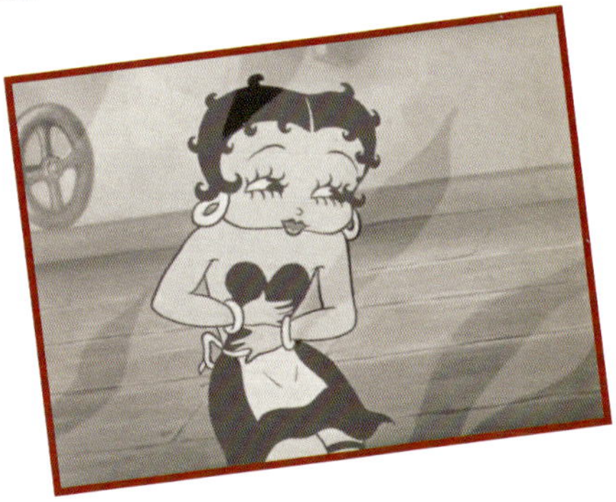

Yet group conversations are limited and certainly would have been at this early time. So, the natural process of laughter became an extension of group conversation. If we think about it, laughter may have been the first chat room. By laughing, an individual could signal their participation in the larger group conversation without actually being involved. Kinda cool.

So, not only did laughter serve an important role in the development of human societies, it was and remains today one of the healthiest things we can do for our mental and physical well-being.

The Language of Laughter

Okay, okay—it's no secret. We love to laugh. It gives us a sense of freedom and relief. It allows us to momentarily forget our problems, difficulties, and pain. It makes us feel good, it's just plain fun, and we have so many choices!

We can snort, whoop, or shriek with laughter. We can howl, giggle, and scream with laughter. We can chuckle, chortle, and cackle with laughter. We can crack-up, split our sides, bust a gut, roll in the aisles, guffaw, roar, cachinnate, crow, belly laugh, and nearly drop down dead and die with laughter. And, love every single minute of it!

Laughter is, indeed, a universal language. It's recognized and practiced all over the world. It's a basic human response that breaks through the cultural boundaries that divide so many of us. It brings people together. It's an essential nonverbal form of communication. And, it's very hard not to laugh when someone next to you is.

Yet, there's a lot more to laughter than what we see on the outside. Are you ready to see what happens on the inside?

Laughter on the Brain

Did you know that we actually have a term for the science and study of laughter? Well, we do. And it's called *gelotology*, which if you ask us is a pretty funny word in and of itself.

Now, what this science tells us is that when we laugh, it involves nearly our entire brain. This is odd because most mental activities just involve one part of the brain or the other. For example, the left half of our brain is the academic hemisphere that's connected to things like logic, language, reasoning, math, and science. The right half of our brain is the artistic hemisphere responsible for creativity, imagination, and intuition.

Let's add to these two hemispheres our frontal lobe, which is involved in social and emotional responses and our occipital lobe, which processes visual signals. Then we have the motor sections connected to physical movement and, of course, our entire limbic system responsible for emotions, including our amygdala, which if you remember is our courage center.

So, different parts of our brain are responsible for different mental and physical functions. Right? But when we laugh our entire brain joins in the fun.

Within seconds of being exposed to something possibly funny, a huge electrical wave runs through our cerebral cortex, moves to the left hemisphere of language, goes to the frontal lobe of emotional responses, travels on to the right hemisphere of artistic creativity, fires up the neurons of the occipital lobe for sensory processing, triggers the motor sections, and sparks the entire limbic system, including the hippocampus, thalamus, hypothalamus, and our very own amygdala. Wow! And, you thought it was just a laugh.

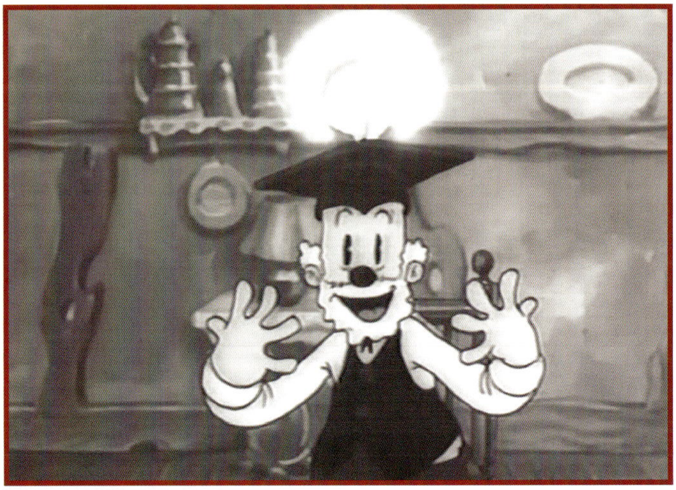

Here's the really fun part. When we laugh and all this activity takes place in our brain, our neurotransmitters jump into high gear. All of our "feel good" chemicals and endorphins, including that dynamic duo of serotonin and dopamine, are released into our system. We feel happy. We feel positive. We feel on top of the world.

Our mood is improved, our outlook becomes rosy, our thinking becomes clear, and our emotional well-being becomes enhanced.

> "WISH ME COURAGE AND STRENGTH AND A SENSE OF HUMOR. I WILL NEED THEM ALL."
>
> –ANNE MORROW LINDBERGH,
> AUTHOR AND AVIATOR

THE THEORIES BEHIND THE FUN

Yep, in addition to all this science we actually have theories as to why and when we laugh. So, just in case you've ever wondered about this, here we go.

The Incongruity Theory

This first theory suggests that we humans are used to logic and order in our lives. We gravitate to those things with which we are familiar. We like and expect our surroundings and the situations in which we find ourselves to be normal and without variation. Accordingly, when two things occur that just don't go together or when an element of surprise is created, our brain senses the "mismatch" and naturally begins to think something humorous is in the air. It's all about expecting one thing and being surprised by another. This sets up an unexpected "turn of events" that the brain finds interesting, enjoyable, and possibly funny.

The Superiority Theory

This interesting concept states that we tend to laugh at something scary or silly when it's happening to someone else. We can afford to laugh at the situation because we are removed from it. Most television sitcoms, for example, are based on this type of humor. We watch the antics of others knowing they're going to fall, get in trouble, reveal a secret, or drink straight gin instead of that expected glass of water. We find this funny but only because we're not involved or affected by the situation. We think we're smarter and wiser. We would never be in the same situation or make the same mistake.

The Relief Theory

Okay, this is one we all know. As humans, we find it hard to watch a situation unfold where it looks like the outcome will be bad, painful, or disappointing. Anticipation in this form is extremely stressful. Think about your favorite thriller movie, for example. Just when the suspense builds to a breaking point and you simply can't bear to watch anymore, one character will suddenly say or do something really funny that cracks us up and makes us laugh. The tension is released and we can relax again, sit back, and enjoy. It's a smart and well-crafted mechanism used extensively in all types of media. And, it's one we often use in real life as well to deal with stress and uncertainty. In other words, laughter takes the place of a huge sigh of relief—comic relief, that is.

In the 1930 classic cartoon *Mysterious Mose,* a very early Betty Boop and her faithful sidekick Bimbo find themselves in a creepy house of shadows, unexplained events, and phantom voices. By morning they can't wait to leave it all behind as they lapse into a welcome, albeit nervous, touch of humor.

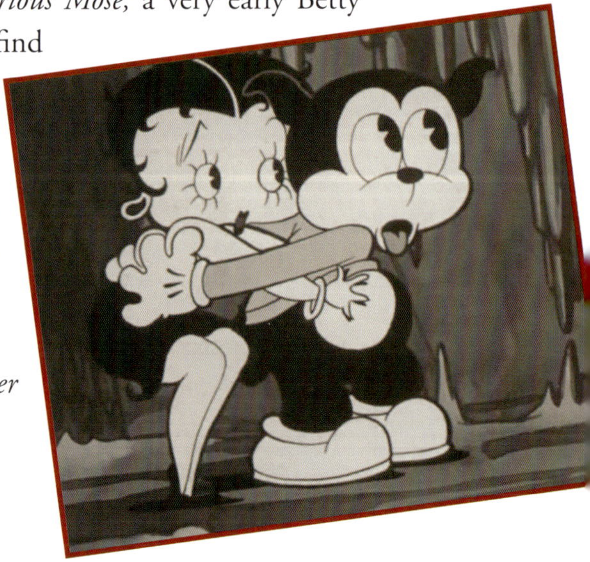

On some dark and stormy night under
the Tempest Moon,
If someone whistles, "Booooooooo"
That's Mysterious Moooooose.

And, don't forget. We don't have to laugh out loud. We don't even have to chuckle under our breath. Because, humor has another important component to it. And that, friends, is a smile.

THE POWER OF A SMILE

Just like it's steadfast companion laughter, a smile can do so much not only for us, but for those around us. A simple smile can transform who we are, what we're feeling, and how the world perceives us.

Every time we smile, we launch a private party in our brain. You see, a mere smile activates another chemical reaction similar to the one we experience when we laugh. Little party-poppers called neuropeptides begin to fire. Our fabulous neurotransmitters and endorphins, including serotonin and dopamine, begin to surge through our neural pathways.

Just like laughter, smiling makes us feel good. It improves our mood and calms our nerves. It makes us feel more positive and hopeful. All those little endorphins help us manage our stress and actually reduce the hormone cortisol, which is the culprit that creates our stress in the first place.

We feel more comfortable.

It's human nature to want to keep things the same. To avoid change or risk. Strangely, smiling decreases this need. Even in very awkward situations a smile can reduce tension and make us feel cozy and comfy.

We appear more trustworthy and approachable.

Science tells us that smiling improves our credibility and makes us seem more understanding and empathetic. We seem nicer. After all, would you rather talk to a person who frowns and appears angry, or to a person who radiates a flashing and friendly smile?

We become more attractive and look younger.

A smile not only looks good on you, but it suggests that you're easy-going, personable, and happy with yourself. And, a smile can make us look at least three years younger because it naturally exercises and lifts our facial muscles, plumps up our face, and reduces the appearance of frown lines. Great to know!

And the really great thing about smiling is that *it doesn't have to be genuine*. Even if you're having a terrible day, everything is going wrong, you feel awful, and the last thing you want to do is smile—do so anyway. Force yourself if you have to. Because the simple act of flexing the facial muscles in a smile position actually tricks our brain into thinking its happy. Really! All our feel-good endorphins will begin churning in our brain. We won't have a choice but to feel better in spite of a difficult day. It's just like flipping a switch!

You know, some people think humor is genetic. Apparently, we humans possess a gene called—wait for it—*5-HTTLPR*. And it's believed that those of us who have a shorter 5-HTTLPR gene are quicker to laugh at funny things and situations. In contrast, those of us with a longer gene are a bit slower to laugh and appreciate the absurdities of life.

But even so—and even if we didn't grow up in a household where laughter was common or a sense of humor was a part of daily life—we all can *learn* to be more humorous by simply doing something fun. Just look at Betty. She always finds a way to have fun!

THE PRINCIPLE–
Get Active and Tickle Your Funny Bone

Betty's Inspiration: Adding a little fun and humor to your life is easy. Anyone can do it!

Read a Funny Book, Watch a Funny Movie, or Binge Your Favorite Sitcom. Revisit cherished comic strips, uplifting short stories, or collection of jokes. Watch cartoons! Betty can certainly recommend a few. The belly laughs are just waiting for you.

Go to Karaoke Night or Visit a Comedy Club. Honestly, have you ever watched a non-singer sing and not laughed? Have you ever listened to a comedian and not at least smiled? These activities are designed to provide a good time and bring enjoyment to everyone. And by the way, about that karaoke—the act of singing itself is uplifting and mood-enhancing.

Watch Baby Animal Videos. After all, there is simply nothing cuter than a bunch of fluffy, goofy little furballs wandering around doing their thing. Adorable and heart-warming. Try YouTube and other online sources, or search your TV guide for suggestions.

Tell a Joke or Two. In fact, set aside time each day to share a joke with family and friends. Even if you don't fall down laughing, a few smiles will get your feel-good chemicals churning.

Join a Laughter Yoga Class. No kidding! This yoga is performed without any reason to laugh whatsoever. Yet, after a few stretching and breathing exercises designed to encourage a sense of playfulness, you'll find yourself smiling and laughing the class away.

Don't Forget to Play. It's simply not possible to play with your child or your pet without laughing, smiling, and feeling good. Child and animal antics never fail to bring a little light-heartedness into our lives.

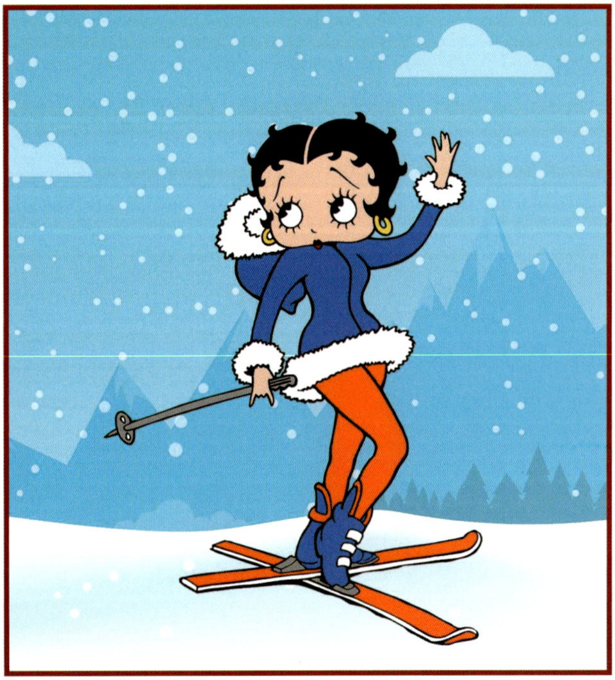

And, if all this wasn't enough good news, there's another thing about a smile we all need to know . . .

SMILING IS CONTAGIOUS

It's nearly impossible to see another person smile and not smile back. No matter how grouchy we may feel. Why? Because of our complex brain activity, that's why. When we see another person smile—or even see a photo of someone smiling—it activates the area of our brain that controls facial movement and a smile is naturally triggered. How great is that?

All right then. We have a pretty firm grasp on just what a sense of humor really means. We understand the importance of laughing and smiling. We know what happens to our brain when we laugh and smile. And we know a good laugh or a bright smile can improve everything from our mood, to our mental functioning, to our sense of well-being. But, there's a lot more to it than that.

THE MORE HUMOR, THE BETTER THE HEALTH

Laughing, smiling, and exercising a sense of humor are three of the most powerful things we can do—and some of the most effective tools for living a happy and productive life.

And while we know this terrific trio makes us feel good, there's a lot more going on than meets the eye. For instance . . .

When our brain feels good, we become smarter, wiser, and more capable people. Our "feel good" chemicals help reduce our mental stress, calm our minds, and balance our emotional well-being. And this creates a chain reaction that has far-reaching benefits of which you may never have thought.

Spontaneity Increases

A little bit of humor literally gets us out of our head. We forget about our troubles and problems suddenly seem far away. When the burden of everyday difficulties eases, we become more connected to our "inner child." Our actions become more "spur of the moment" in nature and we become much better at "winging it" when necessary.

Inhibitions Are Released

The acts of laughing and smiling allow us to drop our expectations of ourselves and the way we interact with the world. Humor paves the way for us to express our true feelings. Fear of rejection, rebuke, or ridicule disappears. And, we act in a way we choose rather than in a way we believe others expect of us.

Negative Emotions Hit the Highway

Anger, resentment, jealousy, and regret have a hard time expressing themselves when we're laughing and smiling. We become less defensive and less critical of others. When we're having a good time, we lose interest in judging others or worrying about the inequalities and injustices of the world around us.

Creativity Surges

A sense of humor opens the door to different and divergent thinking. Remember, we have our entire brain participating in the fun. With all those neurons firing our thoughts become more imaginative and innovative. Our ability to solve problems increases. And if that weren't enough, our memory even improves!

Perspectives Shift

Humor allows us to see things in a new and different way. It's a lot like looking at the world through those "rose-colored" glasses we've all heard about. Our environment becomes less threatening. We're better able to accept new ideas and make new connections. We are less overshadowed by circumstance and more likely to see situations in a realistic light rather than an imagined one.

Moods Get a Boost

Exercising our sense of humor tells our brain we're happy. Our stress hormone cortisol decreases. Our feelings of anxiety and stress are reduced. When we begin to see things in a more light-hearted way, the dark shadows fade away and we become more resilient to the trials and tribulations of daily life.

Decision Making Improves

Humor breeds a positive outlook and a terrific good mood. All this optimism increases our personal feelings of accomplishment and self-confidence. Doubt and discouragement disappear. We become more flexible in our thought process and more decisive in our decision making.

Brain Power Pops

When our brain is fully engaged in laughter and smiling, it's operating at full throttle. Every neuron fires up and becomes excited and active. This mental exercise actually improves our ability to focus and concentrate. It allows us to process information more effectively. It creates a "mindful" environment, which strengthens our neural pathways and sharpens our mental chops.

> "SMILE IN THE MIRROR.
> DO THAT EVERY MORNING AND YOU'LL START TO SEE A BIG DIFFERENCE IN YOUR LIFE."
> –YOKO ONO, MULTIMEDIA ARTIST AND PEACE ACTIVIST

But wait! There's more! Now, let's see what happens to our *physical health* when our funny bone is tickled.

Our Immune System Becomes Stronger

Not only does a laugh or smile reduce our stress hormones, each also increases the fabulous little antibody cells that fight infection and illness. Mirth increases the production of our T cells and B cells, which attack the bad guys in our body like harmful viruses and cancer-causing agents. They fight disease and help our bodies heal from injury and trauma.

Our Heart Is Protected

A good sense of humor can lead to a healthy heart. Humor gets our heart pumping and laughter is a great cardiovascular workout. Laughter increases the flexibility in our blood vessels and lowers our blood pressure. It can help protect us from heart attacks and strokes. And, the benefits of one good laugh can last up to twenty-four hours!

We Burn Calories

No joke! Just ten to fifteen minutes of laughter a day can burn up to forty calories. Laughter is great exercise. Anything from a giggle to a gut-buster engages large areas of body muscles in a good workout. Our facial, shoulder, back, and arm muscles all contract and expand with a good laugh. Our diaphragm and abdominal muscles work so hard they sometimes hurt from the exertion. Never knew laughing could tone your abs, did you?

Pain Is Reduced

We know that laughing and smiling both release endorphins that reduce stress and boost our immune system. But endorphins also are nature's very own personal painkillers. Endorphins change our perception of pain. What's more, each time we enjoy one big belly laugh we can remain pain-free for up to twenty minutes.

We Breathe Easier

A good laugh strengthens our respiratory system and increases our lung capacity. Even a small chuckle pushes oxygen through our lungs that enables us to exhale longer and breathe deeper, pushing life-giving oxygen to every body cell and organ.

"YOU HAVE TO HAVE A SENSE OF HUMOR ABOUT LIFE TO GET THROUGH IT."
–KESHA, SINGER AND SONGWRITER

OUR *WHAT* ON LAUGHTER?

Chakras, that's what. Okay, this sounds like a strange thing, right? But actually, many people today believe that our body is composed of not just the physical attributes that we see like our arms, legs, hands, and feet. But they also believe our body contains hidden "energy portals" that are found literally from our heads to our toes.

A chakra is a Sanskrit word that means "wheel." According to Ayurvedic philosophy, we have seven different chakras aligned in our body. The first Root chakra is located at the base of our spine, the second Sacral chakra is in the lower abdomen, and the third, fourth, and fifth Solar Plexus, Heart, and Throat chakra are located in the, you guessed it, solar plexus, heart, and throat. The sixth Brow chakra is found right between our eyes and the seventh Crown chakra is at the top of our head.

Tracee Dunblazier, certified grief counselor and author of *Master Your Inner World: Embrace Your Power with Joy*, believes that there are three different kinds of laughter that interact with four different chakras.

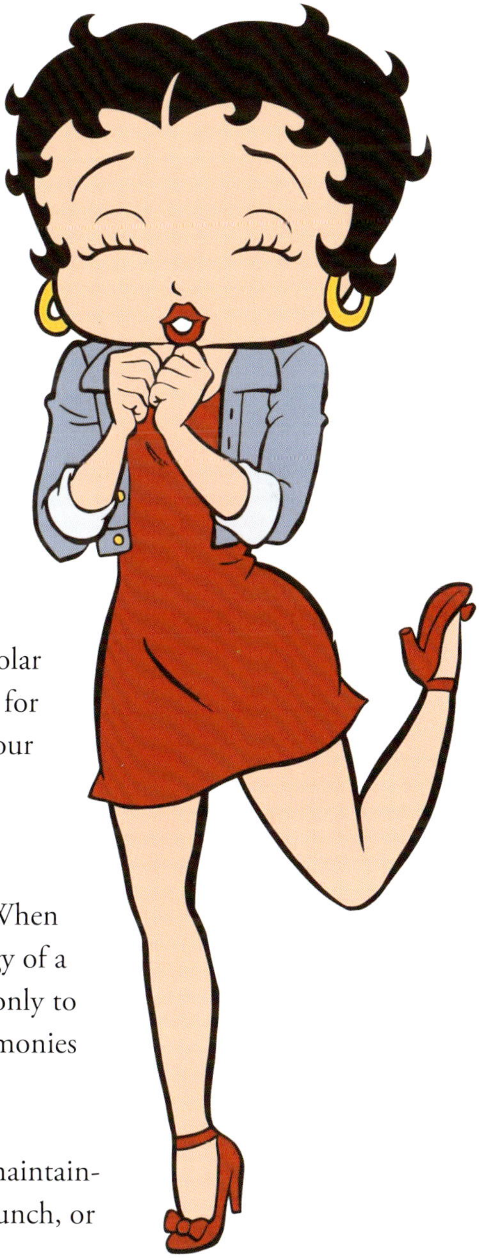

The Chortle

This type of laugh is expressed more on the inside than on the outside. It's centered in the head and deep in the throat, which activates the Throat chakra and improves our flow of communication.

The Guffaw

This one is centered in the belly where it activates the second and third chakras, the Sacral and the Solar Plexus. This laugh is believed to be responsible for increasing our creativity as it affects our will and our desire to succeed.

The Chuckle

And, the amiable chuckle is centered in the heart. When the Heart chakra is triggered, we create more energy of a peaceful nature. The heart itself is opened up not only to our higher self but to the higher energies and harmonies of the universe as well.

Such a nice thing to know, right? And by the way, maintaining our humor can be as easy as having breakfast, lunch, or dinner.

THE PRINCIPLE–
Eat Your Way to Good Humor

Betty's Inspiration: Eating good food not only tastes great and keeps us healthy, but it also nourishes our sense of humor.

Fantastic Fish. Certain varieties of fish are loaded with essential oils called omega-3 fatty acids. This compound has been shown to have the ability to alleviate several mental disorders, including depression and schizophrenia. Sardines, mackerel, and wild salmon added to our weekly diet will improve our disposition and boost our sense of humor.

Nutritional Nuts. Here we go again—more omega-3 to the rescue! Just a handful of cashews, almonds, or walnuts a day will help keep our mental outlook bright and our emotions balanced. We'll feel more positive and we'll be able to see the light at the end of any tunnel.

Tantalizing Tea. Hey now. We all know that a cup of hot tea on a hectic day is soothing and satisfying. Why? One reason is that tea contains friendly flavonoids that stimulate our brain to produce feelings of well-being and relaxation. Chamomile and green tea are great for maintaining a good mood and a great sense of humor.

Fabulous Fruit. The flavonoids don't stop with tea. Citrus fruits like oranges and grapefruit are loaded with them. They keep us feeling good and the antioxidants in citrus protect us from fun-robbing illnesses and diseases.

And Chocolate! A bite or two of dark chocolate each day helps our brain produce that dynamic duo of "feel good" chemicals serotonin and dopamine. Add to this a little methylxanthine and we have a recipe that fights depression, keeps our emotions balanced, and helps us maintain a sunny disposition.

Let's face it. The benefits of humor just don't stop. And when we put all this together, imagine how humor can affect our personal and professional lives. From the bedroom to the boardroom, humor can diffuse difficult situations, put others at ease, heal rifts, build camaraderie, boost productivity, prevent burnout, and supply energy on the most demanding of days.

Humor brings more joy, pleasure, and fun into our lives. It's so much more than just an escape from sadness or pain. It's a powerful tool that leads us down a path on which we can find new hope and greater meaning in our lives.

> ". . . THERE IS NOTHING SEXIER THAN LAUGH LINES."
> –ISLA FISHER, ACTRESS AND AUTHOR

DID YOU KNOW?

Betty Boop's signature voice—Mae Questel—also was the talent for two other classic cartoon characters, Olive Oyl and Little Audrey.

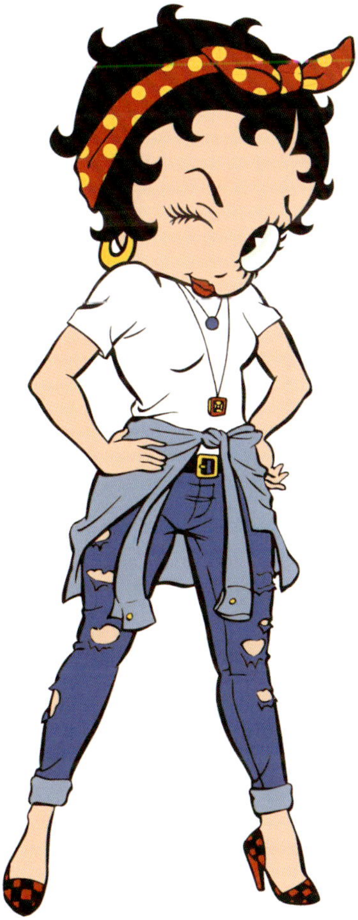

"NEVER
PASS UP THE
OPPORTUNITY
TO SMILE."

Chapter 9

Health—Our Ultimate Wealth

"When you have your health, you have everything."

This is an adage we've all heard most of our lives. Yet, is it really true? Do we really have *everything* if we have our health?

Actually, we beg to differ a bit. We may not have everything when we have our health, *but we have the foundation* to make everything and anything happen. When we're healthy, there are no physical or mental obstacles that keep us from engaging fully in our life. We have the energy and the ability to work hard, think clearly, and pursue our dreams and goals. So, we prefer to say that when we have our health *anything* is possible!

Now, health itself is a rather complicated, multi-layered phenomenon. It can be defined as physical, mental, and spiritual well-being. It can be referred to as a resource for living a full and complete life. It can encompass a good diet, exercise, and adequate sleep. It not only refers to the absence of disease, but also to the ability to bounce back and recover from disease. Good health includes coping strategies, emotional balance, a positive outlook, and a multitude of other factors.

Yet, when most of us hear the word "healthy" we often think first in terms of physical vitality and stamina. We think in terms of "lean and mean" and "no pain, no gain." And for many of us, including Betty Boop, this means *exercise.*

In the 1936 classic cartoon *Betty Boop and Little Jimmy*, Betty is obsessed with "getting in shape" and exercising her way to health. She uses a variety of complicated machines, creating hilarious results that in the end, have Betty throwing up her hands, laughing at herself, and looking for an easier way to achieve her goals.

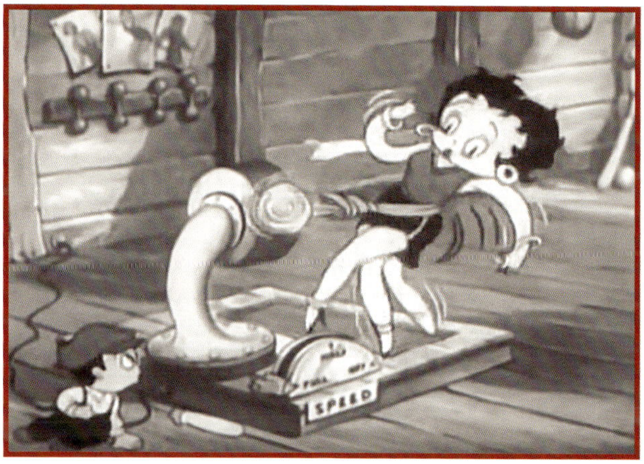

PHYSICAL BENEFITS OF EXERCISE

Exercise has been a part of human life since the prehistoric ages. After all, we had to be strong athletes in order to run long distances, find shelter, hunt, and gather.

Then around 10,000 BC, we moved from our hunter/gatherer stage and began to cultivate agriculture and domesticate animals for sustenance, a lifestyle that demanded a bit less of us in terms of physical endurance.

And as human innovation advanced, physical strength and athleticism were not quite as important as they had been.

In fact, this is when the concept "exercise is medicine" began. Also known as EIM, exercise is medicine gained momentum as our lifestyles became more domesticated and our natural activity levels decreased.

Way back in ancient Greece, the father of modern medicine Hippocrates, wrote the first prescription for exercise for a patient suffering from consumption—better known today as tuberculosis.

In China, a Han Dynasty physician named Hua To prescribed "frolic exercises" for his patients that mimicked the actions of deer, tigers, bears, monkeys, and birds, believing these movements delayed aging and removed disease.

And around 600 BC in India, concerned that people were sleeping too long and eating too much, the physician Sushruta also prescribed exercise because "diseases fly from the presence of a person habituated to regular physical exercise."

Not only was exercise established as a form of medicine, but it also became a pursuit of fun in and of itself.

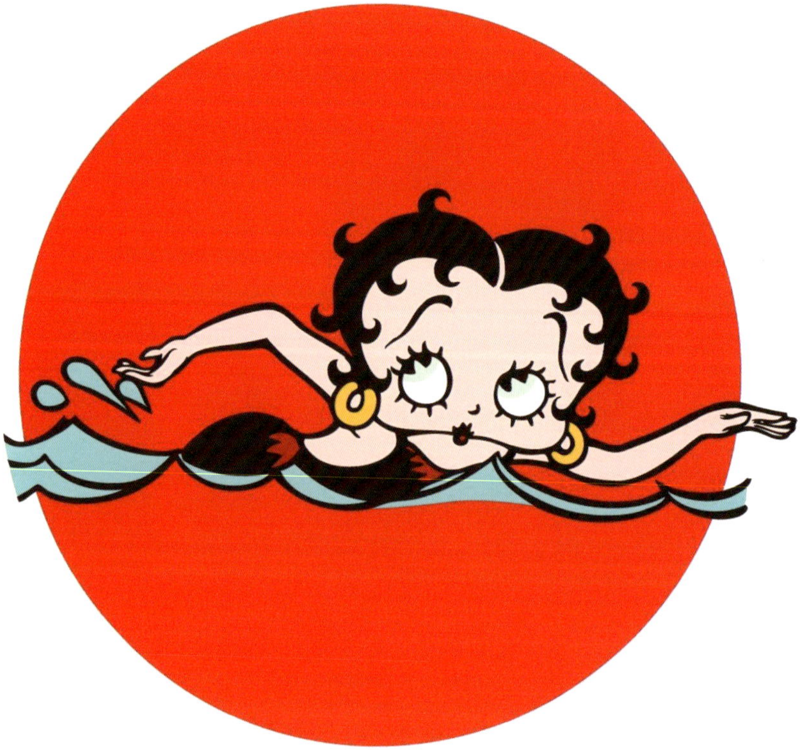

EXERCISE AS SPORT

It was the philosopher Confucius who was so worried about the physical inactivity of the people in ancient China that he encouraged physical activity purely for fun. Kung Fu was the first physical fitness program developed as an "extracurricular" activity. And, with this also came the first sports of wrestling, badminton, and swimming.

Today, of course, physical exercise is one of the cornerstones of a healthy lifestyle. Over the last century, as the modern world emerged and the Industrial

Revolution took place, people everywhere became accustomed to a more sedentary way of life. Diseases such as diabetes and heart disease became more prevalent and leaders and physicians around the world recognized the need for physical fitness as a part of one's daily activity. And, nowhere was this need recognized more than in the lives of women everywhere.

Remember, during the last century women just didn't get out as much as men. Women were more often found in the home, caring for families, cleaning and cooking. Not that this isn't hard work. It is extremely hard work!! Yet, the *perception* of women at the time was one in which we stayed at home and therefore, didn't engage in outdoor activities or physical exercise.

Now, what's really great about exercise is that it comes in many forms. We don't have to be world-class athletes or gold-medal-winning Olympians to get and stay in good physical shape. We don't have to spend full days in the gym body-building or all weekend running marathons. All we have to do is *move.* And, this is something we can do just about anytime and anywhere in many different ways.

> "I'M SO UNFAMILIAR WITH THE GYM, I CALL IT JAMES."
> —ELLEN DEGENERES, COMEDIAN, ACTRESS, AND WRITER

In fact, much of what we already do throughout the day counts as physical activity and enough exercise to reap a bunch of great benefits!

THE PRINCIPLE–
Keep Moving

Betty's Inspiration: Exercise doesn't have to be strenuous to be effective.

It Doesn't Have to be a Chore. Housework can be a wonderful opportunity to exercise. Vacuum the rugs. Do those three loads of laundry sitting in the hamper. Wash those windows. Rake the leaves. Know you are treating your body to a great workout every time housework calls.

Get Used to Taking the Stairs. It's true almost every building in the world has an elevator or escalator, but climbing stairs when you can will make a world of difference in your physical well-being and keep your heart happy!

Park in the Farthest Spot in the Lot. When safety is not an issue, leave your car far enough away from your destination so that you have to walk to and from. It's another great way to sneak some exercise into a busy day.

Don't Forget to Stretch. Simple stretches while standing or sitting at a desk will prevent stiffness and keep our muscles flexible. Raise your arms. Lunge from side to side. Flex your legs. Roll your neck.

You Don't Have to Run a Marathon. Take a walk instead. Even a ten-minute walk around the block will open your lungs, lower your blood pressure, strengthen heart muscles, and improve your cardiovascular health.

"MY OWN PRESCRIPTION FOR HEALTH IS LESS PAPERWORK AND MORE RUNNING BAREFOOT THROUGH THE GRASS."
—LESLIE GRIMUTTER, AUTHOR

So, you bet! Physical exercise is vital for our physical health. It helps protect us from illness and disease. It strengthens our bones, keeps our muscles strong and flexible, and improves digestion and essential body functions. And, of course, it helps us maintain a healthy body weight.

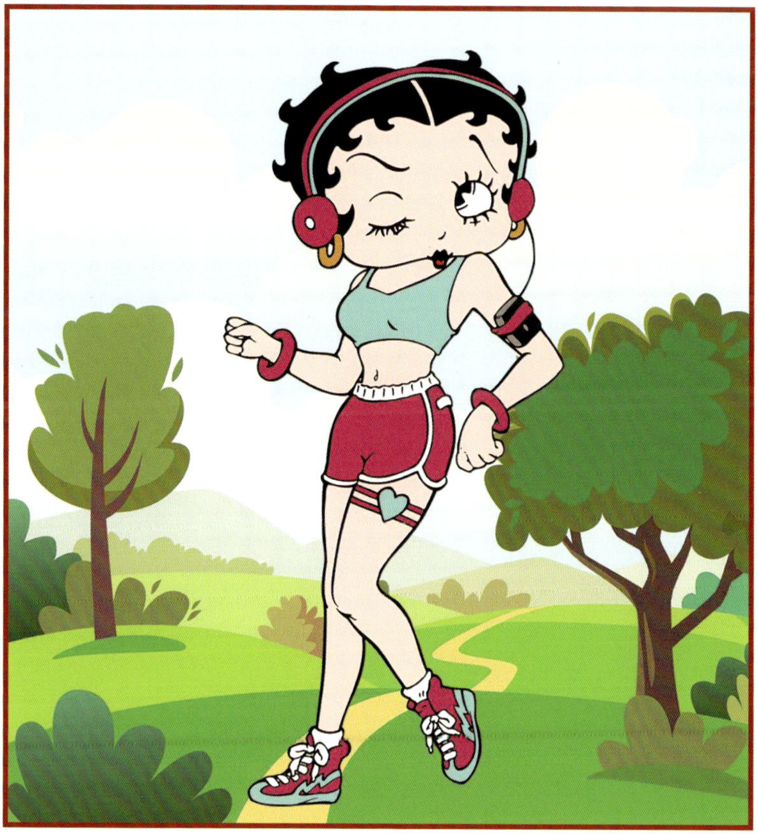

BUT WHAT EXACTLY IS A HEALTHY WEIGHT?

Ladies, this is a tough topic. As women, we are bombarded every day with images of what the female body should look like. And, more often than not, those images depict women who are extremely thin. Moreover, these women are depicted in a way that suggests their popularity, wealth, success, and happiness are all dependent upon the fact that they are thin.

Our culture is constantly sending us signals about our bodies and what we should be striving for. We see images of perfectly photoshopped bodies all around us from fashion models and celebrities to advertisements, clothing catalogs, movies, and television shows. The women making waves, the women in the news, and the women who seem to be the most valued in our society are thin.

And, this is not an accident. This is a deliberate social campaign referred to as *thin-ideal media* in which being extremely thin is highlighted as the best, most desirable, and most attractive way to be.

In fact, if we were to believe the message of thin-ideal media, we all would have to accept that the average modern woman today was about 5'10" and weighed 120 pounds. In contrast, would it surprise you to learn that the average woman is only about 5'4" and weighs about 160 pounds?

Not only is this media message inaccurate, it's damaging. We can't help but feel inferior when we're surrounded by images of unattainable perfection. It makes us feel bad about ourselves and hurts our self-esteem. It makes us feel that we cannot be popular, successful, or happy if we have more body weight and curvaceous curves than the models in the magazines. And this, of course, is nonsense!

Remember, a healthy body weight is not about appearance, it's about *health.*

When we gain weight, we increase our risk for diabetes, high blood pressure, heart disease and stroke, and certain cancers. Yet, when we lose too much weight, we increase our risk for osteoporosis, illness and infection, anemia, nutritional deficiencies, and cardiac problems. The trick is to find the perfect body weight for *you* that will ensure years of healthy living.

Because every woman is unique. Women's bodies come in all different shapes and sizes. And, they all are beautiful!

THE PRINCIPLE– Weight Management 101

Betty's Inspiration: Find your own personal Goldilocks' Zone—not too much, not too little, just right!

DIY BMI. The Body Mass Index is a tool that can help us determine if we have a good body mass to fat ratio for optimum health. It's an easy, popular and well-known measurement technique to see if we are overweight, underweight, or at our perfect healthy weight.

Speak with Your Physician. Ask questions. Express your concerns. Weight management is an important road to travel with someone who has experience with health issues, understands your personal concerns, and knows your health history.

Do It for You. Finding your ideal weight is about you—not your peers. It's about your goals and not the goals of those around you. It's your body and your life. Decide what's best for your optimum health. Then take charge of that decision, run with it, and own it.

Be Realistic. Forget the ads on television. Put away the fashion magazines. Ignore the images of perfect women depicted in the media. Figure out the look that makes you feel attractive. Decide on the weight that makes you feel good. That's what it's all about.

Reward Yourself. Once you reach your personal weight goal, celebrate! Maybe it's time for a new pair of jeans. How about a hairdo to match your new image? Be kind to yourself. Pat yourself on the back. Enjoy your succcss.

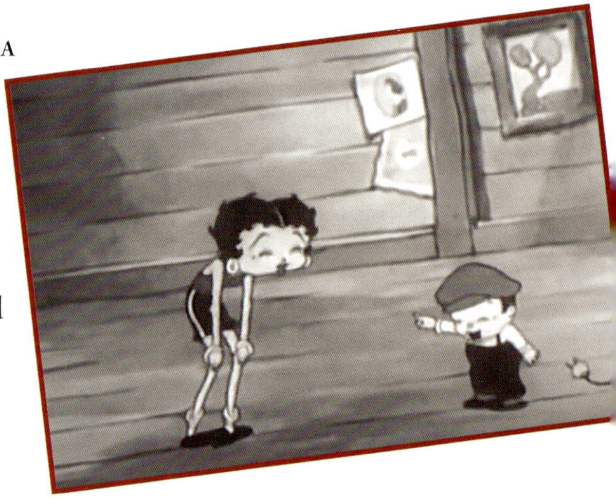

By the Way, Betty Has Never Been a Skinny Girl! She's always enjoyed her curvaceous female figure. Yes, she strives to stay healthy. But just as she learned in *Betty Boop and Little Jimmy,* being skinny isn't the answer. Accepting your body and feeling good about yourself is!

> "THERE IS NOTHING WRONG WITH YOUR BODY, BUT THERE IS A LOT WRONG WITH THE MESSAGES WHICH TRY TO CONVINCE YOU OTHERWISE."
> —RAE SMITH, AWARD-WINNING DESIGNER

MENTAL BENEFITS OF EXERCISE

Now, here's the thing we sometimes forget. Exercise is not just about gaining physical strength, ripped abs, or tight buns. It's about rejuvenation, revitalization, and just plain feeling good. Physical benefits may be the ones we see, but exercise also offers us a bunch of hidden benefits we don't see. Exercise makes our brains happy—just as happy as our hearts, muscles, lungs, and bones.

To understand this, let's go back and revisit our old friend *neuroplasticity.* Remember how our brain works? When we have a particular thought, the brain creates a neural pathway from point A to point B. When we have the same thought again, the brain sends a neural impulse down the same pathway. After doing this over and over again, this thought pattern becomes a rut and it's almost impossible to get out of that rut and think in a new way.

We know that there are mental activities we can do to change the way our brain works. What's great news is that physical activity also can change the way our brain works. Physical exercise stimulates the growth of new blood vessels, new neural pathways, and new brain cells. Exercise helps keep our brain and our thought patterns refreshed and out of the dreaded rut that limits our ability to think and act effectively.

Every time we move our physical body, our wonderful neurotransmitters and "feel good" endorphins like *serotonin* and *dopamine* start churning in our brain. Now, let's add another neurotransmitter known as *gamma-aminobutyric acid*—or *GABA* for short. GABA sends messages between the nervous system and the brain. It reduces the activity of our nerve cells allowing our brain to relax. This reduces our feelings of depression and fear.

Physical exercise also helps protect our *telomeres*. These little guys are parts of our body cells that over time, become shorter. Short telomeres indicate aging and cell damage. Yet, regular physical activity protects our telomeres and prevents them from becoming unusually and dangerously short.

Exercise also helps eliminate stress and anxiety. When we engage in physical activity the level of our stress hormone *cortisol* drops. This allows our bodies to relax and our minds to be calm.

SO, WHAT DOES ALL THIS MEAN?

It means that exercise can improve our memory, boost our good mood, increase our ability to think clearly, fight depression, decrease fear, stress, and anxiety, protect us from mental disease like Alzheimer's, and ensure a healthier and longer life. *Whew!*

Physical and mental well-being are joined at the hip, so to speak. And, exercise will enhance not just the physical attributes of health, but the mental ones as well.

Yet, there are many other ways in which we can enhance and expand our mental and emotional well-being. Activity is important. But so is inactivity. Just as we need to plug into our lives with regular activity, sport, and physical endeavors, we also need time to unplug from our lives.

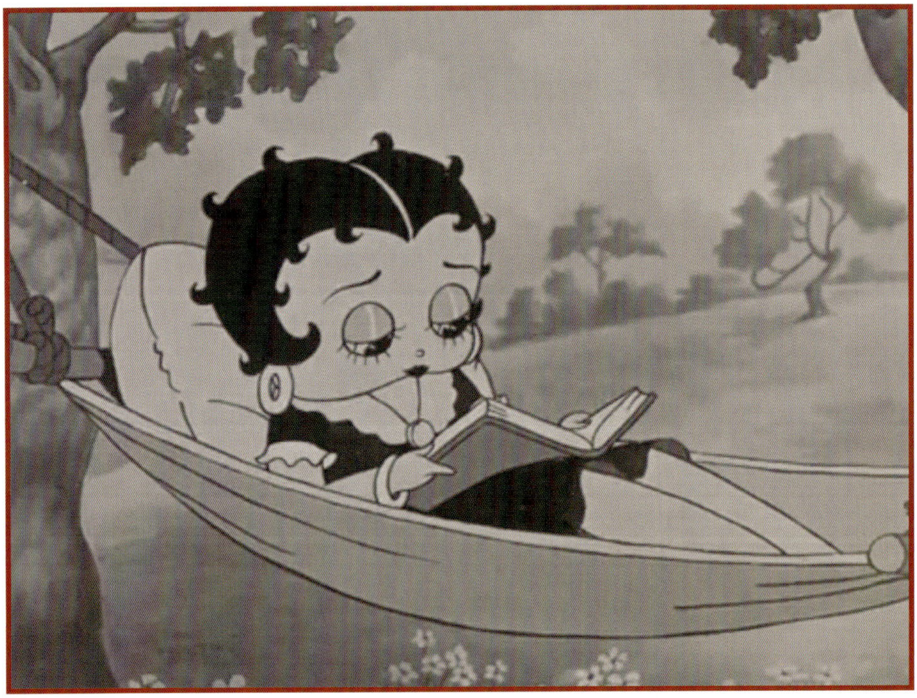

HEALTH IS ABOUT FINDING BALANCE

No one is busier than Betty. From dancing and singing on stage, to running an inn, working in a restaurant, volunteering at an animal shelter, traveling to exotic lands, racing cars, being a judge, babysitting, training lions, and running for president—Betty does it all. Yet, she still finds time to rest, relax, and recharge her batteries.

One thing we can all agree on is that we're all busy. Just like Betty, many of us lead a hectic life filled with responsibilities, duties, and chores. We have massive to-do lists every day and find ourselves running from morning to night. Lots to do, places to go, people to see, and we can't waste a minute! At least, that's the message we receive from the modern world in which we live.

You see, activity is dependent on rest. The *quality of our activity* is determined by the *quality of the rest* we receive. In fact, the power of rest and relaxation may just be the most underestimated things in our life. And this is why!

Rest Repairs Our Bodies

We expect a lot from our bodies and we often push them hard. Many of us tend to push ourselves beyond our physical limitations. We're constantly on the move and even when we feel tired or fatigued, we don't always stop and rest. And, this is a mistake. When our body says it's tired, we need to stop and rest. Rest allows our body to repair itself and recover from daily wear and tear.

Rest Stimulates Our Creativity

We're all vessels of tremendous imagination and creativity. Creativity, however, is hindered when we're constantly distracted by the busyness of life. When our body gets rest, so does our mind. By reducing the external stimulus around us, we decrease our mental noise and chatter. Our mind becomes calm and we can "hear ourselves think." We're more connected with our inner self, which is the source of our creative energy.

Rest Boosts Our Mood

When we rest, we feel better. When we listen to music, read a good book, or watch clouds drifting by, we're not forcing our mind to think in a particular way. We're not trying to solve problems. We're not worrying. Our thoughts determine our mood and when our thoughts are peaceful and harmonious, so too is our mood.

Rest Improves Our Focus and Calms Our Mind

Thinking is hard work. And, mental activity can be just as draining as physical activity. Just as we tend to sometimes push our body beyond its limits, we can push our minds too far as well. Calculating, worrying, making decisions, and solving problems are all exhausting. We have to give our brain a break once in a while. And when we do, we find a little bit of mental peace and quiet actually improves our focus and concentration, which results in more effective action.

Rest Restores Our Energy

We only have so much energy. And, when it's gone, it's gone. Like a car that runs on gasoline, when the gas runs out, the car stops. When we're tired, we need to recharge our batteries and refill our gas tank. Rest revitalizes our nervous system. It activates our spark plugs, gets our wonderful endorphins firing on all cylinders, and gets our engines started!

This all sounds great, right? But, how do we go about shutting off the noise and eliminating all the mental chatter? How do we quiet a brain that's used to being on 24/7? That's a hard thing to do. Especially when we're so accustomed to living a busy life in a hectic world.

Well, Betty has a few ideas about that!

Meditation

This ancient practice is believed to have originated in India. Once considered a discipline for monks and priests, meditation has become a common household practice. There are many forms of meditation yet most of them simply require a person to sit comfortably with the eyes closed. It's not about controlling thoughts—it's about allowing our mind to drift freely without an agenda. This relaxes the nervous system and calms our mind. Forget the iPad, phones, and tablets. Just a few minutes a day of quiet reflection is great for managing stress and relieving anxiety.

Yoga

Okay, you're right. Yoga is a physical exercise. So, what's it doing in the mental exercise section of our book? Well, yoga is a very specialized type of physical activity that has been benefiting women for 5,000 years. Yoga may improve flexibility, balance, endurance, and physical strength, but this passive exercise also shifts our awareness away from the physical sensations of the activity to the emotional sensations that accompany each pose. Our serotonin surges with this mindfulness resulting in an improved mood, a sense of relaxation, and a clear mind.

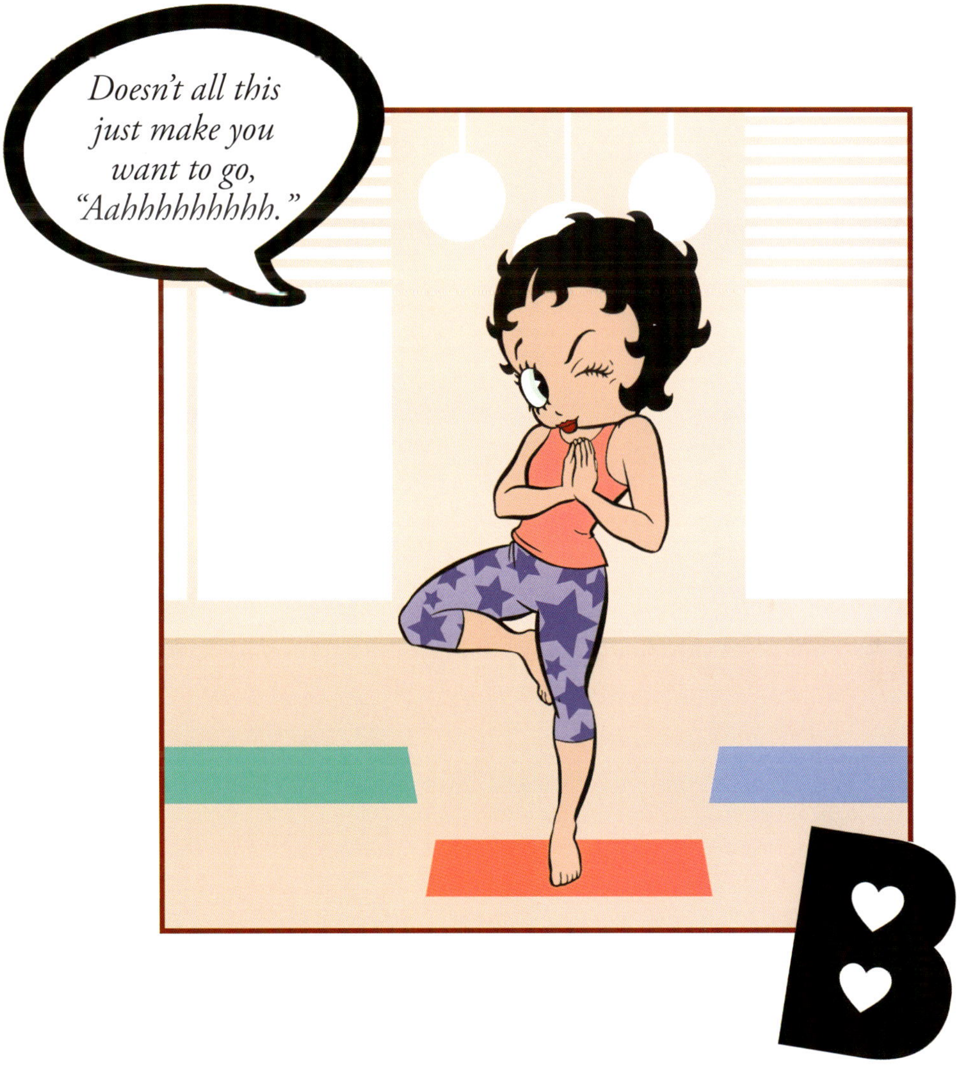
Doesn't all this just make you want to go, "Aahhhhhhhhh."

Creative Visualization

As we mentioned in our chapter on positivity, this technique requires us to form a mental image of something we desire in our mind. The image may involve an object, a situation, or a certain feeling like confidence. For example, if we desire more peace in our life, we would sit quietly with our eyes closed and, perhaps, see ourselves sitting in an open field surrounded by flowers, a summer breeze, and the warmth of the sun shining down. If we're feeling sad, we could visualize ourselves in a situation that makes us happy such as an outing with friends or an evening with a loved one. Doing this will train our neural pathways—remember those?—to actually think we're peaceful and happy. Up goes our serotonin, down goes our stress, and our overall optimism increases.

Deep Breathing

Now, this is very easy to do yet, very powerful. All we do is take deep, slow breaths—in through the nose and out through the mouth. Stretching our arms above our heads as we breathe in will open our lungs, pump oxygen to our brain, and release more of our wonderful endorphins. Our muscles let go of tension, our mental concentration improves, and our mind becomes calm and focused.

You see, the fallacy for the modern woman in today's world is the perception that the more active we are, the more productive we are. Nothing could be further from the truth. We have to balance our activity with rest or our effectiveness and success will be compromised. When we're tired, we may still engage in activity, but we often find ourselves struggling. Tired bodies and sluggish minds do not support effective and efficient activity. When we act from a point of rest, however, our actions have power and strength. This means we'll expend less energy to act and we'll sail through every activity with ease.

DO LESS AND ACCOMPLISH MORE

When our actions flow from a well-rested body and mind, we get more done. Plain and simple. What's more, there are so many little things we can do throughout the day to give ourselves that much-needed break. Never underestimate a little pampering. It's a great way to unplug from a crazy schedule and a super busy life!

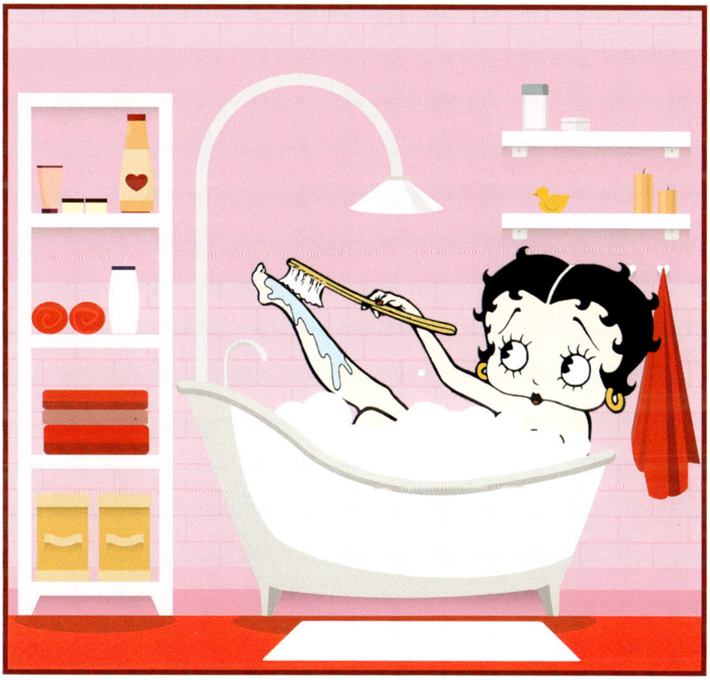

THE PRINCIPLE–
Ideas for Stepping Up Self-Care

Betty's Inspiration: A little me time can go a long way in paving a restful and relaxing day.

Get a Massage. Gentle stroking and kneading of the muscles and tendons can repair damage caused by physical activity. It can reduce pain and eliminate headaches. And, as anxiety melts away, our mind becomes calm and our energy is renewed.

Listen to Soothing Sounds. Your favorite music. Running water. Birds chirping. Rain falling. Listening to nature or beautiful "white noise" is a wonderful way to relax. It can reduce pain and fight depression. It can lower the level of our stress hormone cortisol, restore balance to our minds and bodies, and help prevent illness and disease.

Light a Scented Candle. Not only are candles beautiful, but they're a great way to benefit from a little aromatherapy. The power of scent is an easy way to relax on a busy day. Lavender, lemon, and peppermint do wonders for relieving stress. Sage can improve memory. And, clove, cinnamon, and jasmine can boost our energy.

Take a Warm Bath. The combination of warmth, bodily comfort, and isolation of this simple activity can significantly enhance our mood and our optimism. Our bodies and minds associate the horizontal position of lying in a tub with vulnerability and relaxation. A warm soak relieves pain while inhaling a little steam soothes our nasal passages and reduces inflammation.

A Blanket and a Hot Cup of Tea. Warmth makes us feel good. That's all there is to it. Wrapping ourselves in a comfy blanket is soothing and comforting. Adding a cup of hot tea completes the picture. Green tea in particular will not only relax us but improve our memory and brain function as well.

Gosh! Who knew taking it easy could be so productive?

THE IMPORTANCE OF SLEEP

Of course, our discussion of rest would not be complete without including a few notes and tips on the importance of sleep. Sleep is, after all, the cornerstone of daily rest and vital for ensuring our quality of life and overall well-being.

You see, everything we've discussed so far like meditating, yoga, and self-care are merely supplements to a good night's sleep—they are not replacements.

Sleep remains the foundation upon which all activity is based. In fact, we spend somewhere between one-quarter to one-third of our entire life sleeping. So, let's get it right!

> "SUCCESS, SHE DECIDED, WAS OFTEN A MATTER OF KNOWING WHEN TO RELAX."
> —BARBARA TAYLOR BRADFORD, AUTHOR

Years ago, most people believed sleep was a passive activity during which our bodies and brains were inactive and dormant. Today we know our brains are very active when we sleep and cycle through two different stages known as rapid-eye movement or *REM*—and *non-REM* sleep.

The first stage of sleep is non-REM, which occurs as we transition from our waking state to our sleep state. We then enter light sleep when our heart rate and body temperature drop and our breathing becomes slower. Finally, we enter deep sleep.

It's during this deep sleep that learning and memory are enhanced. It's also the more restful and restorative phase of sleep. During REM sleep, our eyes move rapidly behind our lids. Our breathing becomes rapid, our brains become active, and we begin to dream. This is the learning phase of sleep. Daytime memories are encoded in our brains. We're processing the day's activities so that the next day, our mental abilities and motor skills are stronger.

REM also is the stage that's linked to that feeling of being refreshed in the morning. After all, we know what it's like when we don't get a good night's sleep. It's hard to focus and concentrate. Small problems loom like huge disasters. We get cranky, impatient, and even depressed.

Moreover, our health is compromised. A lack of sleep can lead to high blood pressure, migraine headaches, a compromised immune system, and unintended weight gain.

In the 1935 classic *Stop That Noise*, Betty struggles to get a good night's sleep. But nothing is going right.

Oh, there is no pity
In this great big city,
With this noise, noise, noise!

Of course, we definitely need a little peace and quiet when we're trying to sleep. No doubt about it! But Betty has a few more tricks up her sleeve.

THE PRINCIPLE–
Good Night and Sleep Tight

Betty's Inspiration: Getting your nightly ZZZs can get you through the day with EEEs.

Forget the Exercise. Just before bed, that is. You see, exercise during the day is great for sleeping well at night. But, exercising too late in the day may have the opposite effect. Exercise is a stimulant, which increases alertness and hormones like epinephrine and adrenaline, all of which activate our nervous system rather than calming it down.

Welcome the Dark. Eliminate the light in your bedroom. Close the curtains. Pull the blinds. Shut the bedroom door. Turn your clock around. Shut off all devices. Even the soft glow of LED lights can interfere with sleep patterns and keep you awake at night.

Wear Socks. Warm feet are happy feet. We have lots of little nerve endings that bundle in our feet. Just as bare feet will help keep a drowsy driver alert at the wheel, sock-covered feet in bed will help a restless sleeper relax. Socks cushion the nerves in our feet and prevent neural stimulation that can interfere with sleep.

Find the Perfect Temperature. It's hard to sleep when it's too hot or too cold. Experts seem to agree that 70 degrees Fahrenheit is the most comfortable temperature for sleeping. But everyone's different. So, make sure your bedroom thermostat is set just right for you.

Pass on the Caffeine. Drinking coffee certainly has health benefits. But, consuming any beverage or food that contains caffeine can definitely cramp our style when it comes to sleep. Caffeine stimulates our nervous system and can stay in our system for up to six hours. So, have that cup of coffee or that bite of chocolate early in the day so you can enjoy a good night's rest.

A LITTLE FOOD FOR THOUGHT

Our discussion of health just wouldn't be complete without addressing the importance of food. Food, after all, is a basic necessity of life. All living creatures need to eat in order to sustain energy, grow new body cells, and repair damaged tissues. Food is the fuel that keeps our bodies going strong.

But we need to be careful not to eat just any food. We've all grabbed a bite because we've been hungry. But how often do we grab a bite because we want to be healthy?

No one knows the importance of eating healthy better than Betty. After all, she's worked as a chef and a waitress, she's run a bed and breakfast, and she's always cooking for her friends and family.

But Betty knows that we can't just eat anything and expect to feel well and get through our day with energy and ease. She knows we need the proper balance of the five food essentials: protein, carbohydrates, fats, vitamins, and minerals.

These are the building blocks of a strong and healthy body and mind. And, when we eat the proper food with all the proper essentials, here's what we can expect!

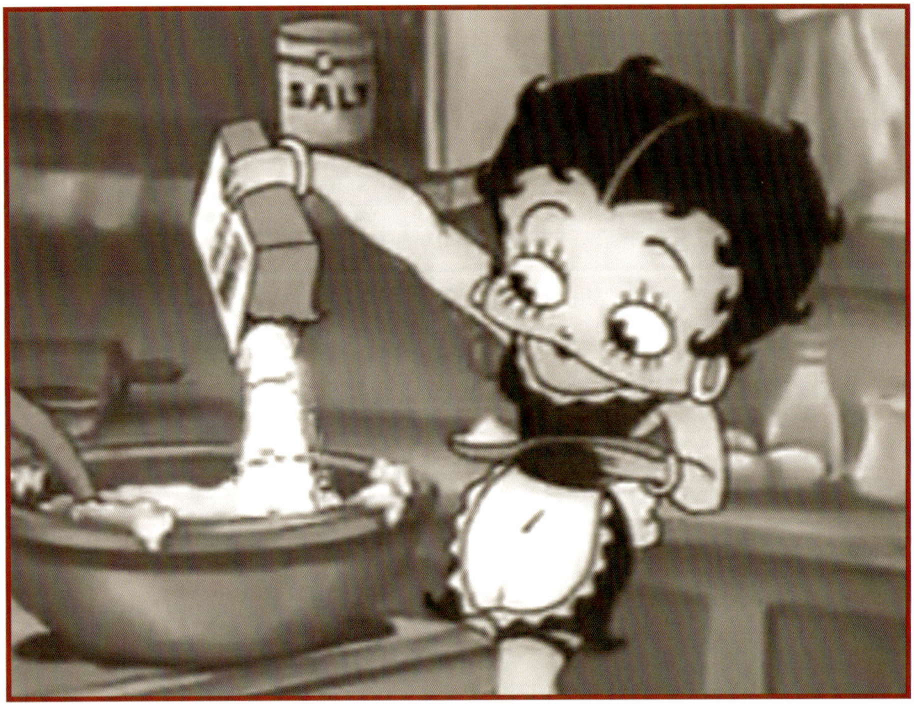

Disease Prevention. Healthy food is like a pharmacy on a plate. Many diseases today are caused by an unhealthy diet. When we eat right, we can effectively fight and prevent a wide range of diseases and illnesses, including osteoporosis, cardiovascular disease, high blood pressure, diabetes, and many cancers.

Weight Control. It's not just the quantity of the food we eat, but also the quality that influences our weight. Now, we want a *healthy* weight. So, we want to consume foods with more fiber and less fat. We want to balance the number of calories we take in with the energy we put out. In this way, our bodies will remain strong and our weight will remain steady over time.

Energy. If you can't pronounce it, don't eat it. Healthy, *whole foods* are essential for providing energy, fighting fatigue, and repairing damaged cells and tissues.

Stick to foods that are unrefined and unprocessed. They contain more of the necessary body-building nutrients and vitamins our bodies need to stay strong and energized all day long.

Mood & Stress. Wonderful whole foods that are high in antioxidants help protect our neural pathways and improve the ability of our brain cells to communicate with each other. This enables us to fight stress, calm our minds, and retain a great mood.

SO, THAT'S *WHAT* WE CAN EXPECT AND HERE'S *HOW* WE CAN DO IT!

Lean Proteins. This includes yummy foods like chicken and turkey breast. Baked or roasted skinless poultry cuts add great protein to your diet without adding extra fat. Eggs and egg whites contain healthy protein while remaining low in calories. Low-fat dairy products will provide protein and boost our energy. And, fish like salmon are wonderful sources of protein and bad cholesterol-fighting omega-3 fatty acids.

> "AS FOR BUTTER VERSUS MARGARINE, I TRUST COWS MORE THAN CHEMISTS."
> —JOAN DYE GUSSOW, PROFESSOR AND ENVIRONMENTALIST

Veggies and Fruits. Many of these pantry staples are loaded with vitamins, minerals, and antioxidants. They help us fight infection, illness and diseases, including many cancers. They're low in calories and high in fiber and flavor. So, bring on the carrots, blueberries, avocadoes, and spinach!

Nuts and Seeds. A handful of walnuts, almonds, or sunflower seeds is not only a great source of protein, but also of fiber and healthy omega-3 fatty acids. They're packed with crunch and flavor. And, just one ounce a day will fight inflammation, heart disease, and keep our weight at its healthy best.

Beans. Legumes are so underrated! Beans, peas, and lentils are wonderful sources of protein and fiber that pack a one-two punch. They help us feel full and keep us from overeating. In soups, sides, and salads, this food choice is versatile and filled with nutritional benefits.

Grains. Carbs get a bad rap because many of us eat the wrong ones. While we want to stay away from the refined carbohydrates in white bread, cookies, and sugary cereals, whole grains are good for us. Whole wheat, whole oats, and brown rice can lower our bad cholesterol levels, decrease our risk for heart disease, and add healthy fiber to our daily diet.

THE PRINCIPLE–
Mindful Eating

Betty's Inspiration: Food can be your new best friend.

Don't Eat Late at Night. That midnight snack can be tempting but it will wreak havoc with your health. We're less active late at night and our metabolism is slower. Eating late will promote weight gain and possibly indigestion. It also will interfere with a good night's sleep—and we certainly don't want that!

Eat Smaller Portions throughout the Day. Instead of eating a big breakfast, lunch, and dinner, try eating five or six small meals throughout the day. A few eggs here, a healthy smoothie there, a small salad anywhere. This prevents over-eating and keeps our energy and metabolism steady all day long.

Chew Your Food Slowly. Give your brain time to catch up with your body. When we eat slowly, we are more aware of how much we're eating and how hungry we are. Once our hunger has been satisfied, it's time to stop eating. This will prevent indigestion, over-eating, and unwanted weight gain.

Dish Up a Balanced Plate. We want a combination of protein, carbohydrates, and vegetables in every meal. Fill one-quarter of your plate with protein, one-quarter with carbs, and one-half with veggies. This creates a perfectly balanced meal designed for optimum physical and mental health.

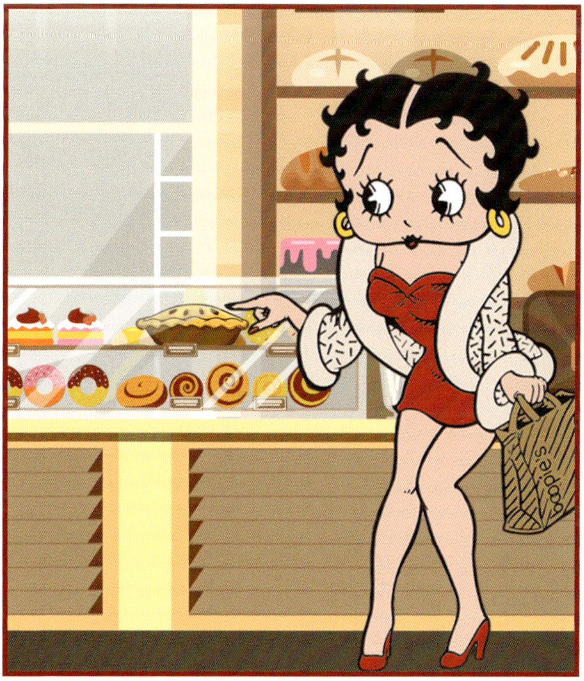

Indulge Once in a While. You really can have your cake and eat it too. Culinary treats are one of life's joys. But don't overdo it. Shoot for a few times a week. Better yet—share that occasional treat with a friend!

Health is not a simple subject because we are not simple creatures. We all have different needs, strengths, and goals. We live in different environments and face different daily challenges. We have different health issues and unique bodies that require different treatments, attention, and care.

Yet, by knowing ourselves, staying informed, and using common sense we can maximize every inch of our potential and live healthy, productive, and exciting lives—just like Betty!

> "IF YOUR BODY'S NOT RIGHT, THE REST OF YOUR DAY WILL GO WRONG."
> –TERRI GUILLEMETS, QUOTATION ANTHOLOGIST AND AUTHOR

DID YOU KNOW?
Betty Boop memorabilia is known as Boopabilia.

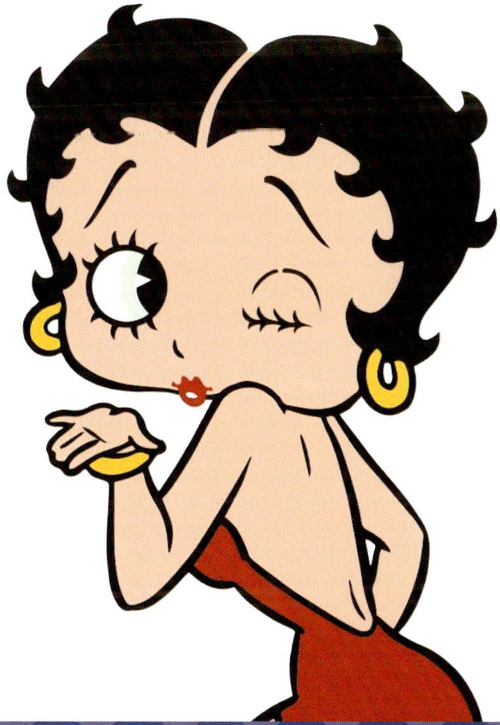

"WHEN WE HAVE OUR HEALTH, ANYTHING IS POSSIBLE!"

Chapter 10

Respect-fully Yours

R**-e-s-p-e-c-t—find out what it means to *Betty*!**

Whether it's the amazing Aretha Franklin belting out a powerful song, or the quiet little voice we hear in our own heart and mind, respect is something we all desire. Respect for our work. Respect for our ideals. Respect for our talent. Respect for our actions. Respect for who we are and the things in which we believe.

> "WE ALL REQUIRE AND WANT RESPECT, MAN OR WOMAN, BLACK OR WHITE. IT'S OUR BASIC HUMAN RIGHT."
> –ARETHA FRANKLIN, SINGER, SONGWRITER, AND CIVIL RIGHTS ACTIVIST

We all seem to know *about* respect and that it's something we all want. But do we really know *what* it is? Can we define respect for ourselves? Do we think we have respect? Do we deserve respect? Do we know how to go about gaining respect?

These are very important questions, indeed. Maybe respect is a little more complicated than we thought? But we do know it's a universal theme that even animated characters have had to deal with throughout their lives.

Our Betty has never had an easy road to follow. She's always been faced with doubts, criticism, ridicule, and that age-old problem of not being taken "seriously." After all, when you grow up in the cartoon world you simply have to try harder to get your message across and establish your place in the universe.

But Betty knows that before we can demand respect from others, we first need to demand respect from ourselves. So, let's begin with this thought and see where it leads us.

SELF-RESPECT

In the 1935 cartoon *Little Nobody*, Betty's beloved puppy Pudgy is tormented and rebuffed by a very beautiful and pampered lady pooch he's trying to befriend. Pudgy is told he's just "not good enough" and he wanders away, tail between his legs, hurt and dejected. Betty, of course, consoles Pudgy and reminds him . . .

Don't you mind if now and then some people laugh at you.
You've just never had a chance to show what you can do.

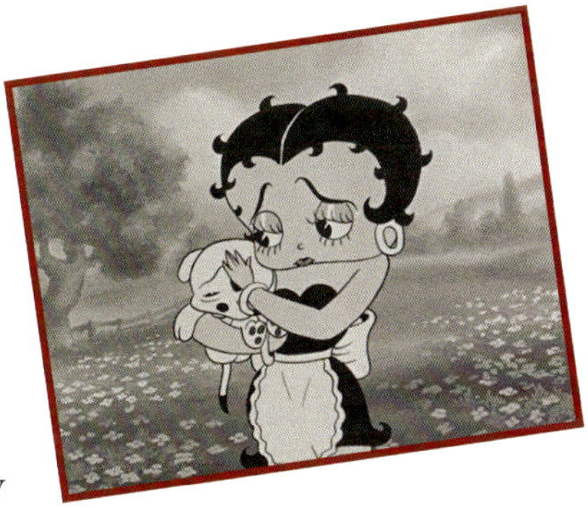

And sure enough, when the pampered pooch falls into a raging river, Pudgy puts his personal feelings of dejection on hold. Believing in himself and his ability to do the right thing, he jumps into the water to save her—gaining admiration and respect from all those around him—especially from himself!

So, what's the lesson? First, as we've already mentioned, we have to believe in ourselves. We have to accept ourselves for who we are—not for what others think we are or want us to be. And we have to accept the entire package. No one is perfect. We all have faults and frailties. We all make mistakes and miss the mark. We all stumble and fall. This is part of the human condition. And this is what we all need to understand and embrace as we develop that sought-after quality of *self-respect*.

"LOVE YOURSELF DESPITE—AND BECAUSE OF—YOUR FLAWS."
—JEWELL PARKER RHODES, NOVELIST AND EDUCATOR

Before we go any further, let's clear something up. Self-respect is not the same as being self-centered, conceited, or narcissistic. It's not about beating someone else in a competition, out-doing the next person, amassing likes and comments on social media, or obtaining lots of cool things and new gadgets.

Rather, self-respect is about a deep sense of personal value and worthiness. It's about loving yourself—warts and all—and being comfortable in your own skin. It's about recognizing your strengths and acknowledging your weaknesses. It's about accepting yourself as you are today—knowing that through hard work and right action—you'll be an even better person tomorrow.

Everything in life is a work in progress. This includes us! If we look closer at Betty and the long road she's traveled, we see lots of changes along the way. Betty is not always perfect. She often finds herself in hot water. Her first choice is not always her best choice. And, Betty sometimes doesn't see the trouble that waits just around the corner.

Yet, Betty is always honest with herself. When she's afraid, she admits it. When there is a problem, she tries to solve it. When someone needs help, she always offers her hand. And these are the enduring qualities that continue to define Betty and the way she feels about herself.

"TO FREE US FROM THE EXPECTATIONS OF OTHERS . . . THERE LIES THE GREAT SINGULAR POWER OF SELF-RESPECT."

–JOAN DIDION, NOVELIST AND JOURNALIST

THE PRINCIPLE–
Establishing Self-Respect

Betty's Inspiration: The road to self-respect may be easier to find than you think.

Be Honest about Your Physical Appearance. Make a list of five things you really like about your body. Make a list of five things you don't like. Now, embrace everything on each list. The good and the less good. Every day, wrap your arms around yourself and send love to every inch of your body and soul.

Be Honest about Your Abilities. List five things you do well. List five things you could do better. Pat yourself on the back for the abilities at which you excel. Make up your mind to improve those things that don't come easily. Be proud of your accomplishments and be gentle with yourself.

Stop Trying to be Normal. In fact, understand that there is no normal. We're all exceptional and one-of-a-kind beings. Each one of us is different from everyone else. Don't try to blend in with those around you. Celebrate the things that make you unique.

Love Notes. You're already learning to be honest with yourself. When you have a good thought or you do a good thing, make a note of it and praise yourself. Write it on a sticky note. Place it where you'll see it on the bathroom mirror, the door of the fridge, in your purse or briefcase. Daily love notes to yourself will remind you of your worth and intrinsic value.

Rely on Your Own Expectations. Don't feel you have to live up to the expectations of others. You know yourself better than anyone else does. You understand your needs, goals, and desires better than anyone else. Learn to please yourself. Trust yourself.

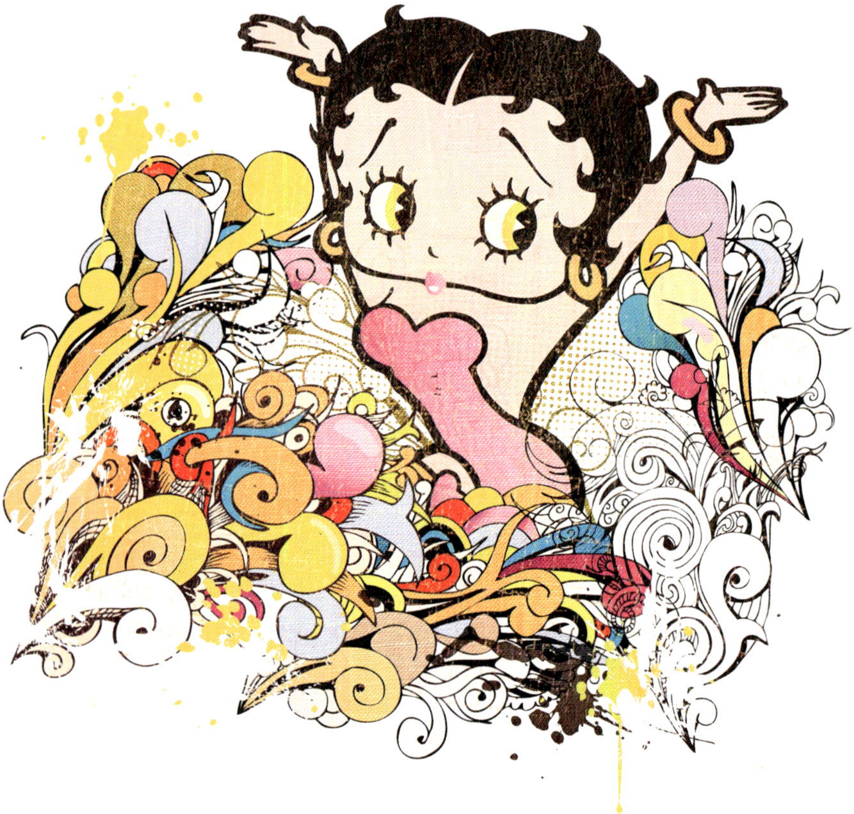

Ultimately, of course, we have to like ourselves. That's really the bottom line on self-respect. And this appreciation of ourselves—this *self-love*—is pretty much unconditional. And, even though it's a concept we've already mentioned, it definitely bears mentioning in relation to respect.

Self-love doesn't depend on success because we'll always have failures to deal with. Self-love is not the result of being better than our peers and comparing ourselves to others, because there will always be someone better at this or that than us. It's not based on how much we have, because there will always be someone who has more.

Rather, self-respect is accepting yourself just the way you are. It's about being your own best friend and having the courage to stand up for yourself no matter what. When we make mistakes, we learn from them and try a little harder the next time. When we fall flat on our faces, we pick ourselves up, figure out *why* we fell and then keep going. When we succeed, we take pride in our accomplishments. Yet while we're patting ourselves on the back, we're also humble enough to know there is always room for improvement.

This attitude is the cornerstone of self-respect. And the really cool thing about this is the great upward cycle: as we develop our own sense of self-respect and treat ourselves with love, kindness and understanding, we're also teaching others how to treat us.

> "JUST IMAGINE HOW DIFFERENT THE WORLD COULD BE IF WE ALL SPOKE TO EVERYONE WITH RESPECT AND KINDNESS."
> –HOLLY BRANSON, PHILANTHROPIST AND AUTHOR

As we become more accepting of ourselves, others become more accepting of us as well. As we recognize our innate value, so do others. As we learn to trust ourselves, so do others. As we learn to embrace ourselves, so do others. As we develop respect for ourselves, so does everyone else. And vice versa! When we learn to respect and feel good about ourselves, we extend all that great energy to those around us. It's a true win/win situation!

STANDING YOUR GROUND

Finding our footing isn't always easy. Betty has had to work hard at that all her life. It takes time to develop a strong sense of who we are. In 1934 when Betty starred in *Poor Cinderella,* she was always trying to gain the respect and admiration of those around her. She worked hard, was always kind, and did her best to be respectful of others.

Of course, we all know how that story ended! Betty won the love and respect of those around her, succeeded in her goals, and realized her dreams. And just like Betty, it's good to know there are things we can do every day to ensure that those around us know we mean business and that we should be taken seriously.

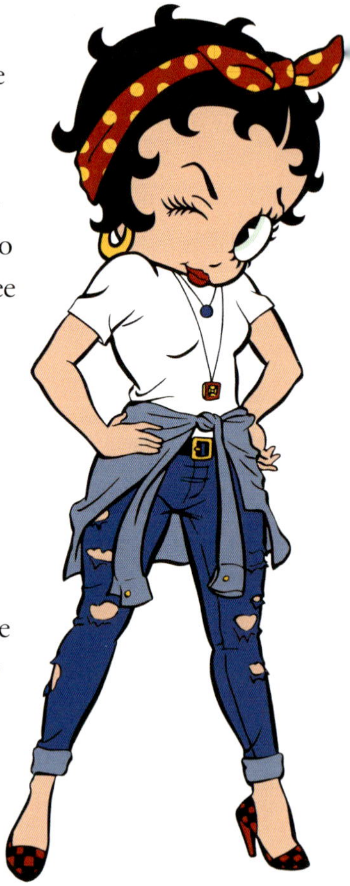

Self-Presentation

We've heard it a hundred times. We only have one chance to make a first impression. And, that impression has to be a good one. Yes, people eventually will accept you for what you offer on the inside rather than what they see on the outside. But in the beginning, others need to see a person who cares enough to act and look their best, and they need to see it immediately. So, dress appropriately. Business attire, for example, doesn't mean jeans and a T-shirt. Make sure your clothes are clean and well-fitting. Comb your hair. Brush your teeth. And, smile. Present the very best version of yourself. Believe us, others will be impressed.

The Power of Body Language

The way we move and hold our body tells other people how we feel about ourselves. When our shoulders are hunched over, our eyes are on the ground or our arms are crossed, we can appear aloof, disinterested, or insecure. In order to command respect and be taken seriously, we need to appear calm, confident, and collected. Stand up straight with your shoulders back, chin up, and walk with purpose. Keep your eyes forward, make good eye contact with those you meet, and lean in slightly to show interest. Use hand gestures instead of crossing your arms or sticking your hands in your pockets. And stay off that smartphone! When you carry yourself well, you carry a message of purpose and strength to all those around you.

Stop Apologizing

For many of us saying, "I'm sorry" has become a go-to phrase. And of course, there are many times in life when we absolutely need to apologize and say we're sorry. But don't let it become a habit. Over-apologizing can be a sign that you're insecure and unsure of your actions and the effect they have on others. When you and another bump into each other simply say, "Excuse me." When you offer a contrary opinion, stand by it rather than apologizing for it. When you have to share unpleasant information, don't deliver the news and then apologize for it. Saying "I'm sorry" every time something awkward or negative occurs is not necessary. Only apologize if you are personally responsible and truly sorry for something. Otherwise, find different ways to communicate your feelings. Say, "Thank you" or "I thought you should know" or "Unfortunately." These phrases convey your concern and respect to others without apologizing for your mere presence.

Getting Heard

Our voice is our calling card. When we speak, we want and need to be heard. Using other people's names when you speak to them will grab their attention. Make sure your voice is loud enough to carry to all those with whom you want to communicate. If necessary, practice exercises to strengthen your voice and improve your articulation. Varying the tone and tempo of your voice as you speak will make your speech more interesting to listen to. Take a breath once in a while. Using pauses while you speak can be an effective way to keep another's attention. Don't overdo the tech talk. Make sure your words are user-friendly and easy to understand.

Assert Yourself

Be proactive. When you're good at something, let people know not by bragging about it, but by taking the initiative. We all have specific skill sets. Take charge of a situation if you know how to help. Volunteer for a job or task with which you have experience. Don't just acknowledge a problem, try to find ways to solve the problem. Speak up with your suggestions and comments. If you feel your ideas are ignored or your comments are interrupted, simply hold up your hand or index finger briefly and say, "I'd like to finish my thought" or "Excuse me, as I was saying." Be polite but be firm. And always respect the thoughts, ideas, and views of others.

THE PRINCIPLE– Gaining and Keeping Respect from Others

Betty's Inspiration: Practice makes perfect in the world of respect.

Own Your Mistakes. No one likes to admit they've made a mistake or that they've been wrong about something. Accepting responsibility for our actions is vital in the world of respect. So, the next time you mess up, recognize it and accept it. When an apology is required, deliver it courageously and without excuses. Not only will others respect you for it, but you'll be amazed at how good a heartfelt apology can make you feel.

Keep Your Word. We often say, "We're as good as our word." If you say you're going to do something, do it. When you make a promise, you're asking another person to put their trust in you. You're also saying to others that you value them and you are willing and able to help them. Following through on your word will increase your trustworthiness among others and gain their respect.

Practice Humility. Take a back seat sometimes. Let someone else shine. Allow others to show what they can do. We don't always have to be in the spotlight. Praising others in their efforts empowers them to do and accomplish more. It demonstrates your respect for their abilities and your confidence in their choices. This in turn, creates an atmosphere of goodwill and mutual admiration.

Control Your Emotions. Losing your temper or overreacting in certain situations can make you appear irrational and illogical. When you're angry, take a deep breath and let it out slowly. Cool down before you have that conversation or meeting. Stay calm and don't get defensive. Avoid accusations like "you always" and say things like "it seems" or "I feel" instead. Others will take notice and appreciate your efforts.

Don't Be Too Nice. We all have to set limitations. Don't agree to do something you don't have time for or you don't want to do. Don't allow yourself to be pulled into someone else's drama. Speak up when you feel mistreated. Stand up for others when it's necessary. Don't be afraid of confrontation, just make sure you remain diplomatic, firm in your stance, and respectful of others. The favor will be returned.

RESPECT BEGETS RESPECT

When our own sense of self-respect develops and we begin to gain the respect of those around us, a *symbiotic relationship* is formed. This means that our interactions with others become mutually beneficial for everyone involved. After all, when we feel good about ourselves it's easy to share that positivity and make others feel good about themselves. And, the benefits we experience from developing this type of relationship are tremendous!

We Gain and Enhance Friendships

Making friends has never been so easy. When we make others feel good, they naturally want to be around us. We become more attractive and accessible. We become nicer. When we come from a non-judgmental place people sense it and want to spend time with us. We develop a more eclectic circle of friends from different backgrounds. Even strangers waiting in the grocery check-out line or the teller at the bank will recognize our ease and want to be a part of it.

We Broaden Our Horizons and Make Better Decisions

Everyone we meet can teach us something new. Meeting people and relating to them in an honest and accepting manner encourages them to open up to us. We gain insights and inspiration from others. We think about the world in new and different ways. We're better able to see the "big picture" when analyzing situations and making decisions. It's easier for us to entertain and enjoy the differences in others and their perspectives when we are confident and secure in ourselves.

We Open Career Doors

Exercising respect in the workplace puts others at ease. Our good feelings about ourselves help transform our workplace into a blessing rather than a burden. Mutual respect reduces stress and anxiety. It creates an atmosphere which encourages team spirit and helps create a fair environment. Promoting these qualities, showing leadership, and demonstrating our ability to motivate others will pave the path to greater success in the workplace.

Others Want to Help Us

Respect not only helps us succeed and achieve our goals, but it also makes others want us to succeed. When people like you, the way you behave, and the way you treat them, they want good things for you. They know you deserve recognition and promotion. Moreover, others are much more likely to help you themselves, do favors for you, promote, and look after you.

Our Reputation Soars

Our reputation always precedes us. When we treat others with fairness, the word gets out. When we value others and their opinions, people find out about it. We become known as a person of integrity and honesty. Remember, our interactions with others never remain isolated. Rather, our behavior is something people talk about and share. Practicing respect ensures those stories about us remain positive.

We Feel Better

Yes, the bottom line is that self-respect and respect from others just makes us feel good. This comes from our own self-love and the admiration we gain from others. We feel more in control of our lives. We feel more capable. We know how to maximize our accomplishments and minimize our defeats. We feel more in touch with the world around us and quite simply, more comfortable in our own skin.

Yet, Betty will be the first to tell us that respecting ourselves and gaining respect from others is just the beginning. Now, we need to expand on this concept and learn how *we show that same respect to others.*

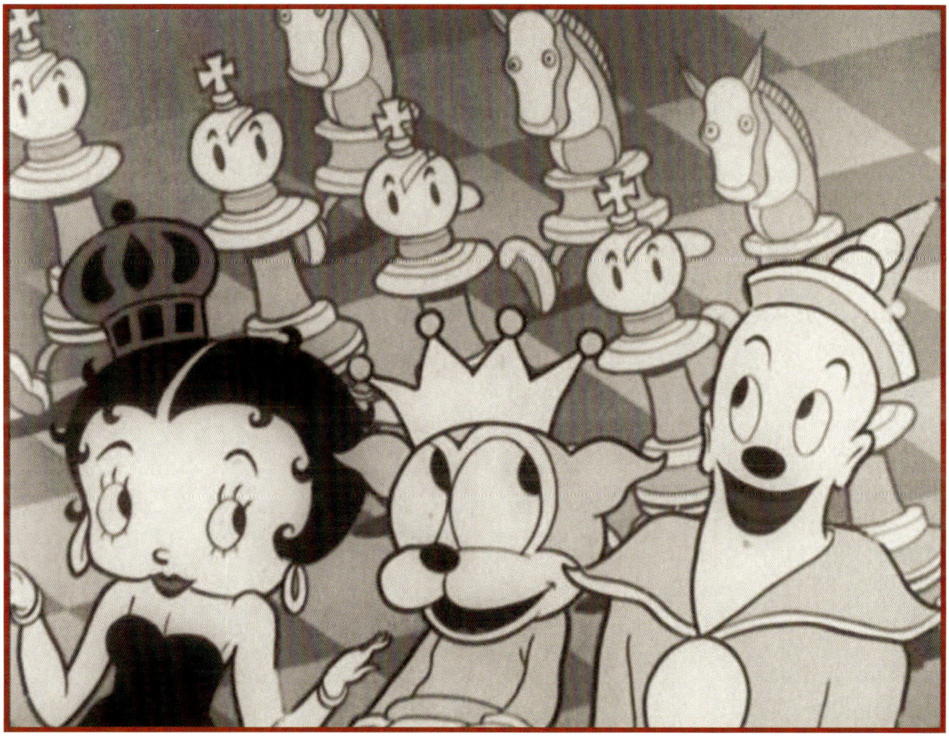

RESPECT FOR OTHERS

All right then. We've established that we can't respect another person if we don't respect ourselves first. Think about it this way—it's kind of like loaning money. We may want to help another person out and give them some money, but we just can't do that unless we have money to begin with. Respect is the same. We can only give it to someone else if we already know what it is and have it inside us. We can only share with others what we already possess.

It really is amazing that once we develop and demonstrate a sense of respect and love for ourselves, people around us tend to treat us in the same way. This non-judgmental manner of treating ourselves and recognizing our own self-worth creates an *aura* of acceptance and understanding that others can't help but notice and emulate.

Fortunately, there are so many opportunities to maintain that aura and share the gift of respect. Every single day we face numerous situations in which we can choose to "spread the love" and treat others as we would like them to treat us.

THE PRINCIPLE– Demonstrate Your Respect

Betty's Inspiration: Simple words and small actions can make everyone feel good.

Offer Congratulations. When someone around you does something well, tell them. When someone else experiences success in their life, pat them on the back. When someone else goes the extra mile, show your appreciation. It's all about making the other person feel good about themselves.

Encourage Others. Life isn't always easy. When you know someone's having a bad time, tell them to keep their chin up. Remind them of all that's going right in their life and compliment them on their accomplishments. Affirm their positive qualities. An uplifting word can make a world of difference on a tough day.

Be Someone's Hero. Does a friend need a babysitter? Is a coworker backed up against a deadline? Sharing your time or offering your advice can mean a lot to someone in need. When you give another person your focus and attention you validate them. *That's* a good thing.

Listen. It sounds easy, but being a good listener can be a tough skill to master. Put your cell phone down and ignore distractions. Look the person in the eye. Tune in to what they're saying and don't interrupt. Everyone wants to be heard and feel that they're being listened to. Showing genuine interest in what someone else has to say can make them feel like a million bucks!

RESPECT OVER RICHES

We've mentioned that when respect is really working as it should, it becomes a two-way street. We feel good. Those around us feel good. It becomes a proverbial love fest! We're not just making this up. These good feelings that emerge are not in our imagination. They're not just wishful thinking. They're not subjective. Rather, these good feelings are real. And, they encompass an objective phenomenon that can be studied and measured by science!

We've already addressed the common misconception that the level of our happiness depends upon the size of our bank account. After all, when we have money, we can buy what we want, we can go out and enjoy ourselves and we don't have to worry about getting the car fixed when it breaks down. And, these are all legitimate observations.

Referred to as our *socioeconomic status,* there is no doubt that having a little money tucked away can make life a easier and a little more fun. But research suggests that the real foundation of lasting happiness has less to do with our overall wealth or success and more to do with something called our *sociometric status.*

Basically, this sociometric status refers to the level of respect and admiration we receive from our peers. Apparently, the more that people around us respect us, like us, and include us, the happier we are. We are social creatures that thrive on the acceptance and nurturing of our friends and family.

In fact, in a series of four different experiments, the results of which were published in the journal *Psychological Science*, researchers found that people with a higher sociometric status—that is, people who were respected within their community, their workplace, or their peer group were just plain happier than people who did not enjoy the same positive social connections. And of these people, even when their wallets were thin, they still felt a deep sense of self-satisfaction and belonging.

On the flip side, people who had more money but not sociometric status simply didn't enjoy the same level of happiness. Rather, these people found financial stability was certainly convenient but not necessarily a source of lasting happiness. And by the way, even with money, when these people felt they didn't have the respect of others, or they lacked satisfying social relationships, or were not considered valued members of their peer group, they were not happy. Plain and simple.

So, it appears the old adage, "Money can't buy happiness" is really true to some extent. Instead, what really seems to matter is the *acceptance* we feel from others, the *admiration* we receive from others, and the *validation* we earn from others. Our perception of happiness is based on the extent and success of our interactions with others as a valuable contributing member of the group.

After all, Betty has never been a woman of financial means. But she has always been a proactive and positive influence in her own life and the lives of those around her. She always shows respect for others. And she's always been an exuberant and positive force for the greater good.

By the way, we've already established that Betty isn't a superhero. She's an ordinary girl just like us who goes the extra mile by taking small steps—not by taking stupendous leaps. And just like Betty, we can all show a little more respect by doing nothing more than being polite and minding our manners. Really!

"I RESPECT EVERYBODY, BUT AT THE SAME TIME,
I CARRY MYSELF WITH AN AURA
THAT DEMANDS RESPECT."
–LIL' KIM, RAPPER, SONGWRITER, AND ACTRESS

THE PRINCIPLE–
Manners Matter

Betty's Inspiration: Minding our p's and q's—a little etiquette is always welcome.

Say Please and Thank You. Such a little thing, but so important. The basic exchange of saying "please" and "thank you" to everyone, everyday, for everything is the easiest possible way to show others you value them and validate their presence.

Let Someone Else Go First. Yes, we're all in a hurry. Yet, try offering another person your place in line. Particularly if that person is older, struggling with packages, or caring for children. Or for no particular reason whatsoever! This simple act can make another person's day while making you feel wonderful. A little respect and recognition. That's what it's all about.

Drive with Care. Good manners extend to the road. Honk when it's necessary, not when you're impatient. Use your turn signals. Keep enough space between you and the other cars. Be careful not to cut another car off. Keep name-calling and hand gestures to yourself. No one needs a hostile environment when they're just trying to get to work or purchase groceries for their family. Good road manners not only show respect for others, but they also help keep us all safe.

Remember to RSVP. Events, parties, and dinners require a lot of planning. The host needs to know how many guests to expect, how much food to prepare, and how many tables and chairs to provide. Always réspondez s'il vous plaît to an invitation. It shows appreciation for your host's time and effort. It says "thank you" even if your response is "no thank you." And, it's a good way to ensure you get invited back!

Hold the Door. Exercise a little patience. It is, after all, a virtue. We're all in a hurry, but stopping and holding a door open for those around us is a class act that will never go out of style. It's an old-fashioned gesture that will always elicit a round of smiles and appreciation.

And while we're on the subject, bad manners exist as well and there are a lot of things that we shouldn't do!

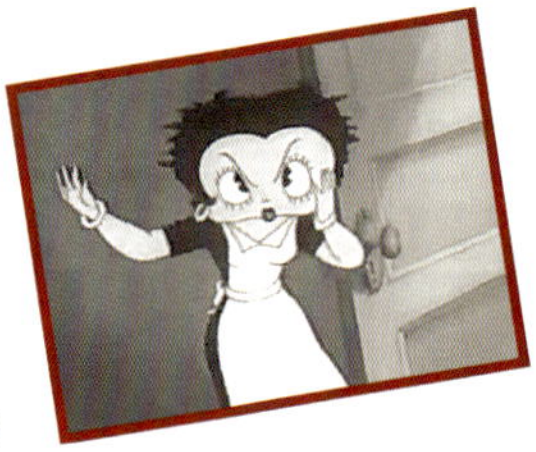

Use that napkin on the table to occasionally wipe your mouth, not to blow your nose. Don't be habitually late. Stop the gossip and excessive swearing. Clean up after yourself. Don't talk loudly. Don't take credit for someone else's work. Chew with your mouth closed. Only comment on another's physical appearance if it's complimentary. Don't ask another to lie for you. Don't swipe someone else's sandwich from the office fridge. Never pick at your teeth, nose, ears, skin or any other body part when in public. Yikes! Need we say more?

"RECOGNIZE AND RESPECT EARTH'S BEAUTIFUL SYSTEMS OF BALANCE, BETWEEN THE PRESENCE OF ANIMALS ON LAND, THE FISH IN THE SEA, BIRDS IN THE AIR, MANKIND, WATER, AIR, AND LAND."

—MARGARET MEAD, CULTURAL ANTHROPOLOGIST AND AUTHOR

SPREADING THE LOVE

And now, it's time to consider the bigger picture. You see, it's not enough to just respect ourselves and those around us. Human beings are not the only form of life on earth. Animals and plants also are living, breathing, seeking creatures as well. And they have as much right as we humans do to be cared for, nurtured, and respected.

Betty has always been a champion not only for her fellow human beings, but for her furry friends as well. In *Be Human,* we've already discussed how Betty stood up to aggression to protect animals that could not protect themselves. Similarly, in Betty's 1937 *The New Deal Show,* she invents new ways to make the lives of all the animals around her better.

> *We have just invented*
> *things to make our pets*
> *contented things.*
> *They all say, "Gee whiz!"*
> *What a wonderful*
> *world this is.*

And no matter where Betty finds herself, she always has time to smell the roses, hug the trees, and appreciate the bounty of nature all around her. Her respect has always extended to her community and the world in general. In fact, Betty was one of the original environmental proponents of recycling, reusing, and repurposing.

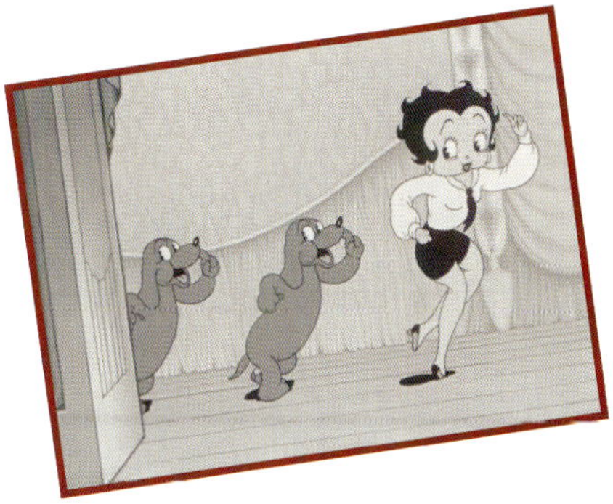

In 1933 Betty's *Crazy Inventions* brought us wonderful new ideas to recycle old items. Everything from shoes, to sardines, to seashells were ingeniously recycled by Betty, her best friend Bimbo, and her devoted Grampy. And in the 1932 *Any Rags?* Betty began her own traveling retail store delivering goods to those who reused and repurposed them in creative and hilarious new ways.

Yet in Betty's world, the perception of respect and being respectful doesn't stop here.

Did you know, in Betty's cartoons nothing is considered inanimate? Everything is alive with feelings, thoughts, ideas, goals, and dreams. Everything has emotions and opinions. Everything shares a sense of humor, the gift of love, and the joy of family and friends.

The clock on the wall has a face that comes to life and speaks the correct time. The front door of Betty's house opens itself with a big smile and a wink. The stones by the lake start laughing and skipping themselves over the water. The broom puts gloves on its spindly hands before it begins cleaning. The dirty dishes have a diving competition into the kitchen sink. The wooden chairs offer themselves to weary guests. The pictures talk, the telephones answer themselves, the pen and pencil dance, and the cars sing to each other as they drive along.

In Betty's 1939 *So Does an Automobile,* Betty becomes a mechanic who tends to the sick and injured automobiles that "run" to her garage for help. Each one has a different problem and Betty has a remedy for everything that ails them.

XOXO

People have engine trouble, like after a happy meal.
People get sick and rundown. So does an automobile.

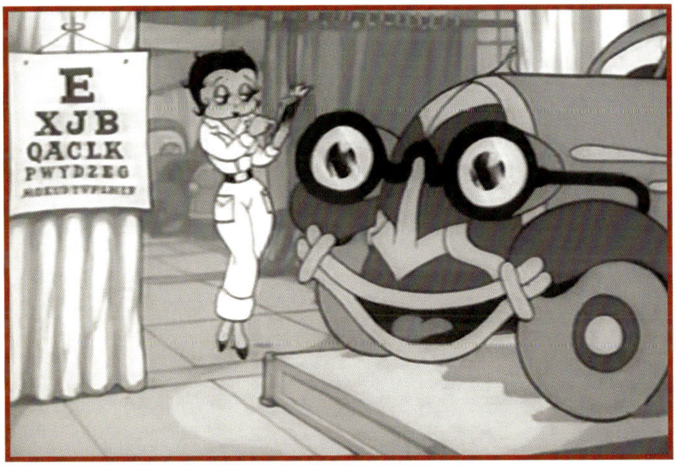

By the way, this concept of seeing *everything* as a living extension of ourselves is not really such a far-fetched idea. If we take a quick look at quantum physics—a quick look, we promise—we see that *everything* from us, to animals and plants, to rocks and Grandmother's china is composed of molecules.

These molecules, of course, adhere to one another in different ways and vibrate at different frequencies. This is why one thing appears as water, another as concrete, and another as your next-door neighbor. So, one theory is that essentially all matter—whether it's animated or unanimated—is at some level the same. Hmmm . . . anyway, it's food for thought. And in Betty's cartoon world, this is definitely the case. Everything is alive and, therefore, deserving of validation and respect.

That's a Wrap!

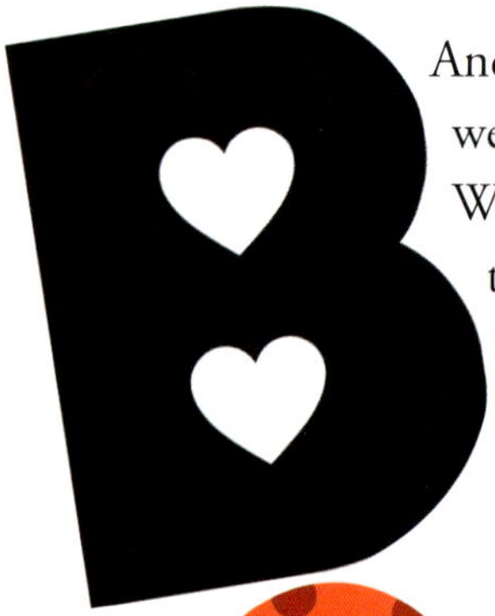

And with that, ladies, girlfriends, and worldly women everywhere, we come to the end of *Betty Boop's Guide to a Bold and Balanced Life*. We hope you've had some laughs. We hope you've learned a little thing or two. And, we hope you've enjoyed yourself along the way. Betty, by the way, has had a blast with you as have we. And, we're so grateful for your company!

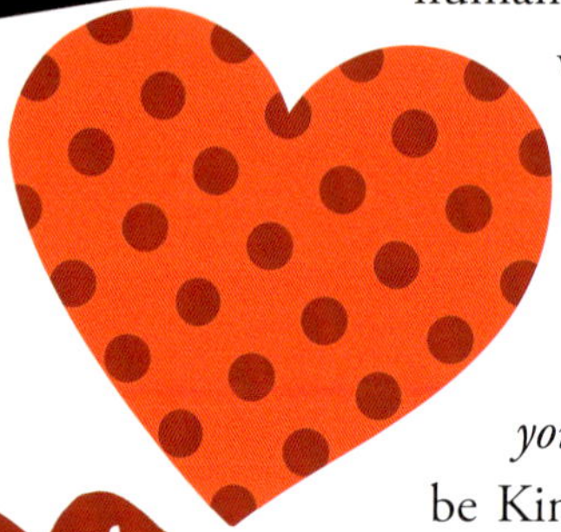

For if anything is clear, it's that the true core values of being human don't really change over time. Betty's struggles, observations, challenges, and victories over the last ninety years are proof of that. Perhaps what people say is true. *"The more things change, the more they stay the same."*

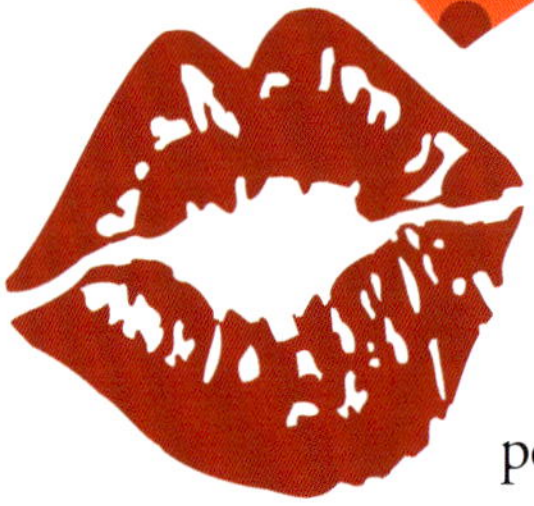

Now it's time for you to get out there and *strut your stuff*! Exercise your Independence, find your Love, be Kind, do it all in Style, remain Positive, move forward with Courage and Confidence, never lose your sense of Humor, take care of your Health and make Respect for all a priority in your life.

You are a fabulous and powerful being packed with potential and possibility. *You* have so much to share and so much to give. *You* have everything you need to succeed in your goals, turn your dreams into reality, and make the world a better place!

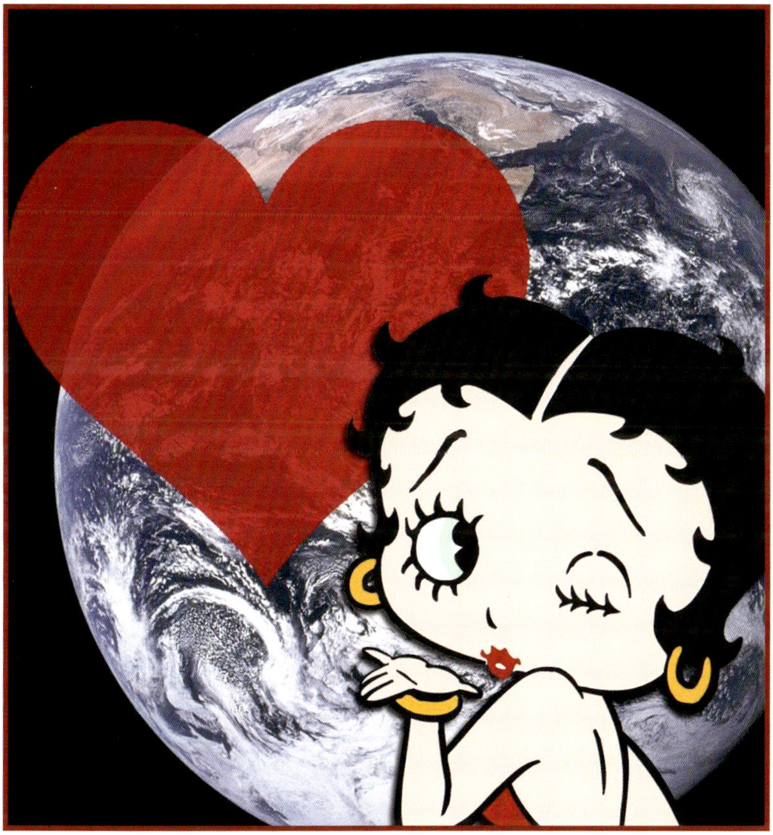

"YOUR LIFE WILL BE WORTH LIVING
IF YOU DO YOUR SHARE.
YOU'LL FIND A THRILL IN GIVING
THAT'S BEYOND COMPARE."
—BETTY BOOP

DID YOU KNOW?
Betty Boop was the first cartoon star to ever be profiled on the Arts and Entertainment Network's acclaimed *Biography* series.

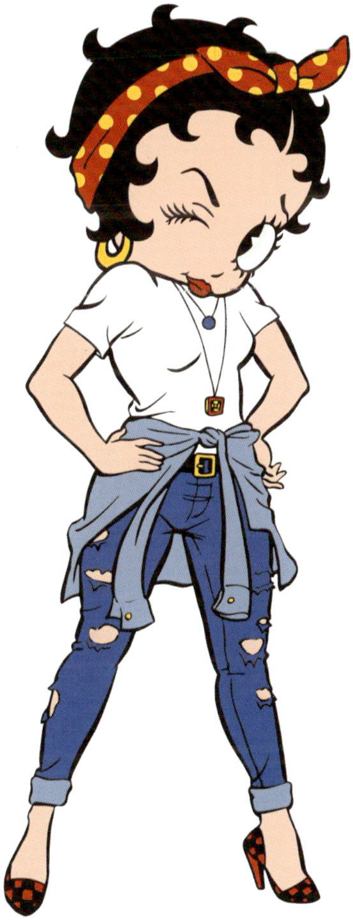

"YOU ARE CAPABLE OF AMAZING THINGS!"

Acknowledgments

To begin, this acknowledgment section would not be complete or possible without first paying tribute to the inspired creativity of pioneer animator and inventor, Max Fleischer, the creator of Betty Boop. It was, of course, Max, his brothers, and the ingenious animators at Fleischer Studios who first brought Betty to the screen and into the hearts of fans everywhere.

Throughout the years, there have been many individuals who have made invaluable contributions to Betty's ongoing success, including Fleischer Studios' General Counsel Stanley Handman, our long-time agents and current colleagues at King Features Syndicate, and their original visionaries Cathy Titus, Ita Golzman, and Frank Caruso.

We'd also like to thank those whose efforts have helped us bring this book to our readers around the world, including Fleischer Studios, Waterside Productions, Inc., Margot Hutchison, Bill Gladstone, Zac Posen, Mark Fleischer, Ron Spencer, Jeni Mahoney, and Jerry Beck.

Of course, we extend a big thank-you to the wonderful folks at Skyhorse Publishing, our editor Leah Zarra, and their entire team for believing in this project and helping us bring it to fruition.

And finally, we send huge hugs and thanks to all of Betty's fans for their unwavering love and support. They are the glue that has kept Betty front and center for decades past—and the promise she'll remain sure and strong for decades yet to come.

About the Authors

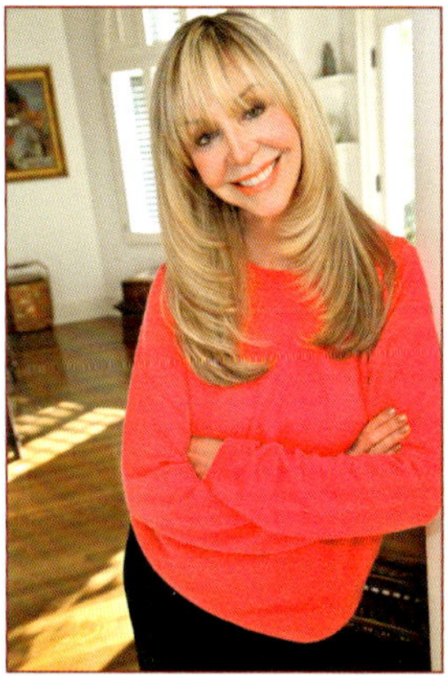

© LEGACY 10 PHOTOGRAPHY

Susan Wilking Horan is an author, attorney, and businesswoman who with her husband Mark Fleischer, CEO & President of Fleischer Studios, and their business partners, has catapulted Betty Boop from the worlds of animation and Hollywood history into the real-life world of Betty fans in 58 countries across the globe. In addition to her accomplishments at Fleischer Studios, Susan is a three-time cancer survivor, a champion of women's health and wellness, an Amazon bestselling author of *The Single Source Cancer Course*, a blogger, speaker, and outspoken advocate for the rights, wellbeing, and empowerment of women everywhere. Visit her online at SusanWilkingHoran.com.

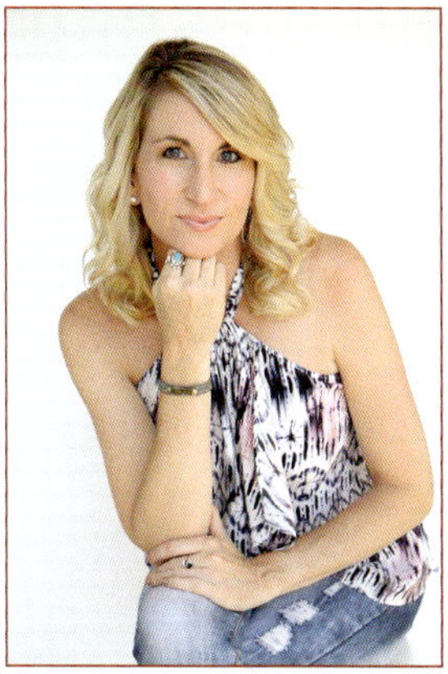

© LEGACY 10 PHOTOGRAPHY

Kristi Ling Spencer is a writer, inspirational speaker, branding expert, and happiness strategist who works to help others create a firm foundation for joy, well-being, and living a magical life. She has been featured in numerous media outlets, including *Women's Health, Reader's Digest*, *Entrepreneur*, *Mashable*, *CNN*, *Fox News*, *Woman's Day*, and *The Huffington Post*. She connects thousands of followers daily on social media with her inspirational messaging. Her acclaimed first book, *Operation Happiness: The 3-Step Plan to Creating a Life of Lasting Joy, Abundant Energy, and Radical Bliss*, was chosen by *Success* Magazine as one of the best books to make you successful. Connect with her at kristilingspencer.com.